LEARNING
Electro
Cardio
Graphy

LEARNING
Electro
Cardio
Graphy

S N Chugh
MD, MNAMS, FICP, FIACM, FICN, FISC, FIMSA

Senior Professor of Medicine
Pt BD Sharma PG Institute of Medical Sciences

and

Pro-Vice Chancellor
Pt BD Sharma University of Health Sciences
Rohtak, Haryana

Eshan Gupta
MD, DM (student)

Senior Resident in Cardiology
GB Pant Hospital
New Delhi

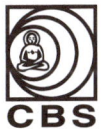

CBS

CBS Publishers & Distributors Pvt Ltd

New Delhi • Bengaluru • Chennai • Kochi • Kolkata • Mumbai

Bhopal • Bhubaneswar • Hyderabad • Jharkhand • Nagpur • Patna • Pune • Uttarakhand • Dhaka (Bangladesh)

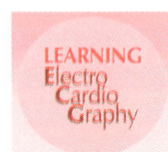

ISBN: 978-81-239-2314-7

First Edition: 2013
Reprint: 2019

Published by Satish Kumar Jain and produced by Varun Jain for
CBS Publishers & Distributors Pvt Ltd
4819/XI Prahlad Street, 24 Ansari Road, Daryaganj
New Delhi 110 002, India.
Ph: 23289259, 23266861, 23266867   Website: www.cbspd.com
Fax: 011-23243014   e-mail: delhi@cbspd.com; cbspubs@airtelmail.in.
Corporate Office: 204 FIE, Industrial Area, Patparganj, Delhi 110 092
Ph: 4934 4934   Fax: 4934 4935   e-mail: publishing@cbspd.com; publicity@cbspd.com

Branches

- **Bengaluru:** Seema House 2975, 17th Cross, K.R. Road,
  Banasankari 2nd Stage, Bengaluru 560 070, Karnataka
  Ph: +91-80-26771678/79   Fax: +91-80-26771680   e-mail: bangalore@cbspd.com
- **Chennai:** 7, Subbaraya Street, Shenoy Nagar, Chennai 600 030, Tamil Nadu
  Ph: +91-44-26680620, 26681266   Fax: +91-44-42032115   e-mail: chennai@cbspd.com
- **Kochi:** 42/1325, 1326, Power House Road, Opp. KSEB Power House
  Ernakulam 682 018, Kochi, Kerala
  Ph: +91-484-4059061-65   Fax: +91-484-4059065   e-mail: kochi@cbspd.com
- **Kolkata:** 6/B, Ground Floor, Rameswar Shaw Road, Kolkata-700 014, West Bengal
  Ph: +91-33-22891126, 22891127, 22891128   e-mail: kolkata@cbspd.com
- **Mumbai:** 83-C, Dr E Moses Road, Worli, Mumbai-400018, Maharashtra
  Ph: +91-22-24902340/41   Fax: +91-22-24902342   e-mail: mumbai@cbspd.com

Representatives

• **Bhopal**	0-8319310552	• **Bhubaneswar**	0-9911037372	• **Hyderabad**	0-9885175004
• **Jharkhand**	0-9811541605	• **Nagpur**	0-9021734563	• **Patna**	0-9334159340
• **Pune**	0-9623451994	• **Uttarakhand**	0-9716462459	• **Dhaka (Bangladesh)**	01912-003485

Printed at: India Binding House, Noida, UP, India

Preface

I am delighted to present this book entitled *Learning Electrocardiography* based on my previous publication *Practical Electrocardiography*. Over the years, I have realized that to understand electrocardiography by undergraduate students is becoming difficult because all the books written on electrocardiography are stereotyped. No book is oriented to teach ECG to the beginners. Undergraduate students are more concerned with simple problems of ECG. They want to know the components of ECG complex and their main abnormalities. Based on this concept, I have completely revised the book and kept the title *Learning Electrocardiography*. It mainly stresses on the elementary ECG, abnormalities of PQRS-T complex (hypertrophies, conduction disturbances), simple arrhythmias and myocardial ischaemia/infarction.

In fact undergraduate students are not much interested to learn the ECG in detail because of the fact that ECG is either placed as a spot for interpretation in MBBS examination or asked during *viva voce*. Therefore, they like to go through the book just before the examination. Students want ECG interpretation, in short, just examination-oriented facts. I have chosen those topics which are commonly asked in the examination. I hope this small book will suit the undergraduates/beginners to learn ECG.

I am thankful to CBS Publishers & Distributors for bringing out this book in colour.

SN Chugh

Contents

2. Normal Electrocardiogram   29

3. Conduction Disturbance   43

4. Disturbance of Cardiac Rhythm   71

5. Abnormalities of P Waves, QRS Complexes and T Waves **108**

1 Elementary Electrocardiography

- What does an ECG mean? What are its indications?
- The electrical stimulation of the heart
- Action potentials and waveforms
- The electrical cardiac axis
- The electrical rotation of the heart

WHAT DOES THE ELECTROCARDIOGRAM (ECG) OR EKG MEAN?

It is defined as a graphic representation of the electrical potentials generated in the heart on a paper by surface electrodes. The electrical events are displayed as waveforms in different planes.

Indications or Uses of ECG

The clinical diagnosis is made from the history and physical examination. The ECG being a bedside investigation helps in immediate diagnosis. In some cases, the ECG monitoring is done for management. The uses of ECG are:

1. Atrial and/or ventricular hypertrophy.
2. Myocardial ischaemia and infarction. The success of thrombolytic therapy for acute myocardial infarction is governed by it.
3. It is a gold standard for diagnosis and management of arrhythmias.
4. Conduction disturbance (heart blocks).
5. Myocardial and pericardial diseases.
6. Effects of drugs, electrolytes, poisons on the heart.
7. Detection of efficacy of various cardiac intervention procedures, i.e. angioplasty, bypass surgery, etc.
8. More advanced ECG technology include stress ECG to diagnose asymptomatic coronary artery disease. Holter's

monitoring is used to relate symptoms with ECG and signal-averaged ECG to determine prognosis of arrhythmias. Now-a-days there is an increased use of ECG in pacemaker functioning/dysfunctioning.

Conduction System of the Heart (Fig.1.1)

The heart has a specialised conduction tissue through which impulse travels. It comprises:

1. *SA node:* It generates the pace or impulse due to its intrinsic property.
2. *AV node:* It is a specialised area in the atria at atrioventricular junction.
3. *Bundle of His:* It is a specialised bundle present in the septum.
4. *Bundle branches:* Bundle of His in the septum divides into right and left bundle branches. The left bundle further divides into anterior and posterior fascicles.
5. *Purkinje fibers:* Within the ventricular muscle mass, there are specialised conduction fibers called *Purkinje fibers* which spreads the impulse slowly.

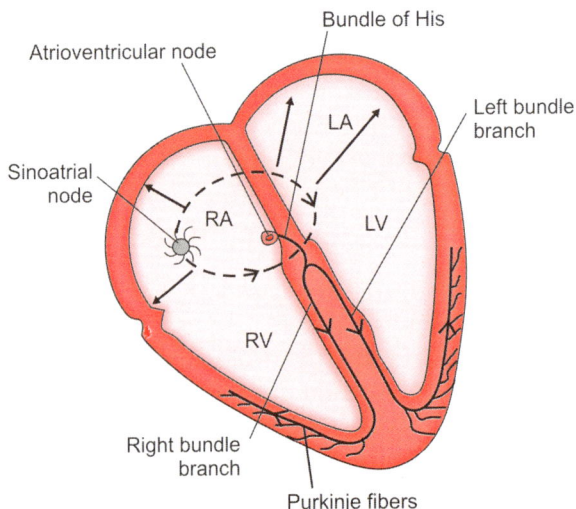

Fig. 1.1: Conduction system of the heart and spread of excitation wave from sinoatrial node to the ventricles is represented by arrows

What does an ECG Complex Indicate?

An ECG complex (P-QRS-T complex) indicates the total electrical events that occur during one beat.

- The P wave represents the atrial depolarisation and repolarisation of atria.
- The QRS complex represents ventricular activation (depolarisation).
- The T wave indicates ventricular repolarisation.

What does an ECG Complex Record?

The ECG complex records electrical impulses from the heart as deflections or waveforms on the graph paper.

Normally, an individual cell is excitable but its activity does not reach to the surface because of a weak electrical potential; but cumulative effect of a group or groups of cells can make electrical potential reproducible on the surface as resultant electrical force or potential which is recorded as deflection or waves.

ELECTRICAL STIMULATION OF THE HEART

How is an ECG Complex Produced?

An ECG complex is produced by electrical conduction of an impulse from SA node to the ventricles.

It involves two processes:
1. Atrial events
2. Ventricular events, e.g. depolarisation and repolarisation (recovery).

1. *Activation of atria (atrial events):* Normally, the SA node (a natural pacemaker) situated in the upper part of the right atrium generates the electrical impulses spontaneously and regularly. The electrical impulses from the SA node travel through three conducting pathways in atria (anterior, middle and posterior internodal pathways) to the atrioventricular (AV) node. These pathways transmit the electrical impulses to the atrial muscle cells which get activated (depolarised) in an organised fashion to produce a P wave on the ECG.

P wave represents atrial activation.

2. *Activation of ventricles:* From the SA node, the impulses reach AV node where a slight physiological delay occurs. From AV node, the impulse enters *bundle of His* which splits into two conducting pathways, i.e. right and left bundle branches. The right bundle branch conducts impulses to the right ventricle via a special network of conducting fibres called *Purkinje fibers*.

The left bundle branch further divides into anterior and posterior fascicles which conduct the impulses to the anterior and posterior portions of left ventricle via the *Purkinje system* respectively. The ventricular activation (depolarisation) produces QRS.

3. *Ventricular recovery:* The recovery or relaxation of ventricles is represented by T wave.

THE ELECTRODE AND THE LEAD SYSTEM

The Electrodes

The ECG lead system consists of 5 electrodes; four for the limbs and one for the chest which is moved at different positions on the precordium. The identification of electrodes is done either by the colour of the electrode (colour coding system) or by the label on the electrode, i.e. RA (right arm), LA (left arm), RL (right leg) and LL (left leg). They are placed above the wrist and ankles or alternatively on shoulders and lower abdomen near the junction of each limb with the trunk. In an amputed limb, it is placed above the amputation stump. The right leg electrode acts as a ground electrode for all the leads (Fig. 1.2).

What is 12-Lead ECG?

A 12 leads ECC is standard and conventional method to record the electrical activity of the heart from 12 different views in two planes, i.e. *frontal* and *horizontal*.

- Frontal plane leads include leads I, II, III, aVR, aVL and aVF. These are called *standard leads*.
- Horizontal plane leads include V_1 to V_6, also called *chest leads*.

Thus 12 leads are classified into two lead systems:

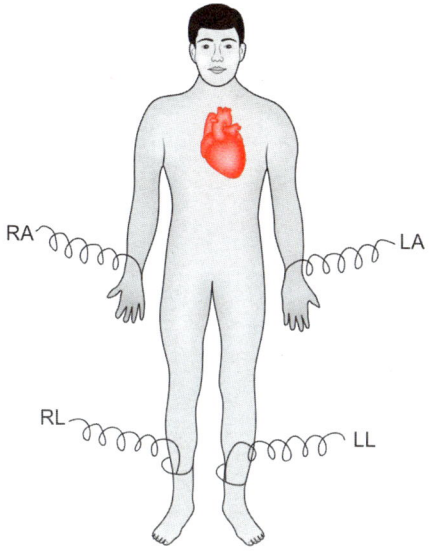

Fig. 1.2: Limb electrodes and their positions. RA = Right arm, LA = Left arm, RL = Right leg (ground electrode), LL = Left leg

1. *Limb leads (bipolar leads):* The bipolar leads require two electrodes at a time to record the tracing; one acts as a positive and the other as a negative electrode. The bipolar limb leads consist of leads I, II and III.

The same bipolar leads are used to form the unipolar limb leads, i.e. aVR, aVL and aVF; where the letter 'a' stands for 'augmented' which means the electrical forces in these leads are enlarged in response to electrically created negative centre.

2. *Chest leads (unipolar leads):* The chest leads are also unipolar leads where either a chest electrode is moved at six different positions or six different chest electrodes are placed at different positions.

These leads are designated by the letter 'V' as V_1, V_2, V_3, V_4, V_5 and V_6. The placement of the electrodes is represented (Fig. 1.3).

V_1 Fourth intercostal space, right sternal border.

V_2 Fourth intercostal space, left sternal border.

V_3 Midway between V_2 and V_4.

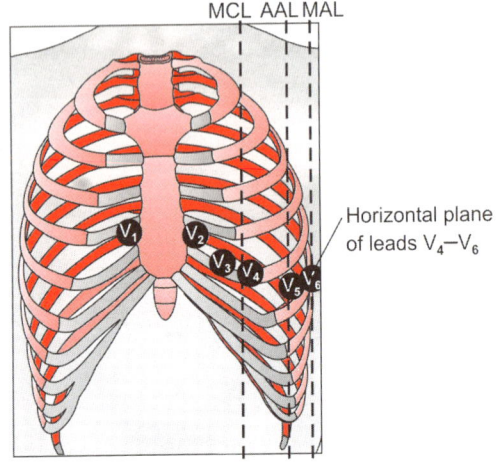

MCL AAL MAL

Horizontal plane
of leads V₄–V₆

Fig. 1.3: Placement of chest electrodes

V_4 Fifth intercostal space, left midclavicular line.
V_5 Fifth intercostal space, anterior axillary line (AAL).
V_6 Fifth intercostal space, midaxillary line (MAL)

The letter V stands for unipolar. These leads need one electrode for recording, hence called *unipolar leads*. This electrode is positive (+) with reference to an electrically created negative centre in the machine which augments the electrical forces.

Note: The same lead system can be used on the right side in a case of dextrocardia or to record right-sided events in a case with pulmonary embolism, right ventricular infarction or right ventricular hypertrophy.

Why are there so many Leads?

Different leads serve different purpose. The 12 leads are diagrammatically presented in Fig. 1.4. The purpose served by various leads is discussed below:

- Leads II, III and aVF are oriented to inferior surface of the heart, i.e. they represent electrical events of inferior surface of heart (Fig. 1.5).

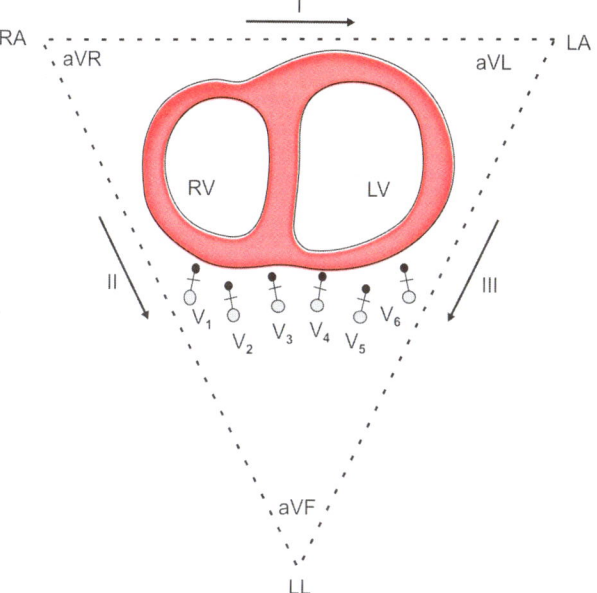

Fig. 1.4: The 12 leads system of electrocardiogram

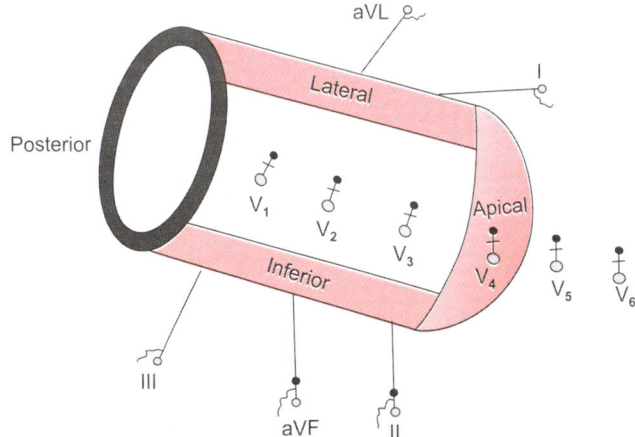

Fig. 1.5: Orientation of various leads to the left ventricle (shown as a cone). Note that there is no lead representing the posterior surface

- Leads I and aVL are oriented to high left lateral wall.
- The lead aVR is a cavitary lead, i.e. records all the negative waves (negative P-QRS-T complex).

- Leads V_1–V_6 are oriented to anterior wall of the heart; leads V_1–V_4 are called anteroseptal leads, leads V_5–V_6 called apical leads and leads V_3–V_4 called transition leads or interventricular septum leads. They represent events of anterior wall of both ventricles.

What is Continuous Monitoring System?

In a hospital, bedside continuous monitoring of ECG is done in CCU (coronary care unit) in critically ill patients. One or more leads may be monitored. A three lead system is used in which one electrode acts as *positive* (+), other acts as *negative* and the third electrode acts as a *ground electrode* (Fig. 1. 6).

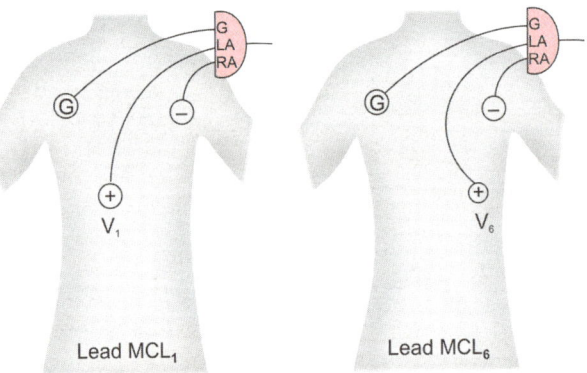

Fig. 1.6: Continuous monitoring system. The connections for modified chest lead MCL_1 and MCL_6 are shown

In this system, one limb lead (I, II, III) may be recorded by placing the electrodes in respective positions while ground electrode is kept underneath the right clavicle. In modified chest lead (MCL) system, one can record any chest lead by just placing the positive electrode in the respective position of that leads, e.g. if positive electrode is placed at V_1 position, then it becomes MCL_1 system and if placed at V_6 position, then called as MCL_6 lead system.

ACTION POTENTIAL AND WAVEFORMS

Each muscle cell in the heart is stimulated to contract (mechanical event) by going through an electrical process (electrical event) called the *action potential*. The action potential curve consists of 5 phases (0, 1, 2, 3, 4). The ECG records the summation of the action potentials of the muscle cells in the atria and ventricles as P-QRS-T waveforms (Fig. 1.7).

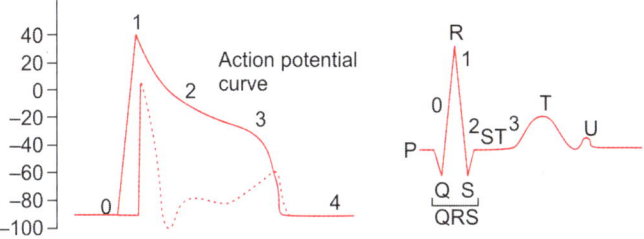

Fig. 1.7: The phases of action potential (0, 1, 2, 3, 4) correlate with the waveforms (P-QRS-T) recorded on ECG (a diagram)

Phases of Action Potential

Resting Stage—Phase 4 (Charged and polarised cell membrane)

Normally, at rest, the cardiac cell membrane has positive (+) charge outside and negative (–) charge inside due to cations. These cations are unable to cross the membrane at rest, hence, no charge flows and the membrane is said to be polarised or charged. This is mainly due to dominance of K^+ inside the cell which leaks slowly at rest and keeps the membrane positively charged outside and negative inside. This resting stage of the muscle is called *phase 4* of the action potential.

Depolarization (Phase 0 action potential)

When a stimulus, say electrical current via ECG machine is applied to the resting cell, it gets electrically activated and flow of ions occurs, i.e. Na^+ moves inside and K^+ moves outside. There is reversal of polarity (the charge on the inside of the cells changes from negative to positive and on the outside from positive to negative) is called *depolarization or phase zero (0) of the action potential* (Fig. 1.8B). Depolarisation being an activation process can be recorded on the ECG as waveforms. Therefore, the P wave on ECG indicates atrial depolarisation and QRS indicates ventricular depolarisation.

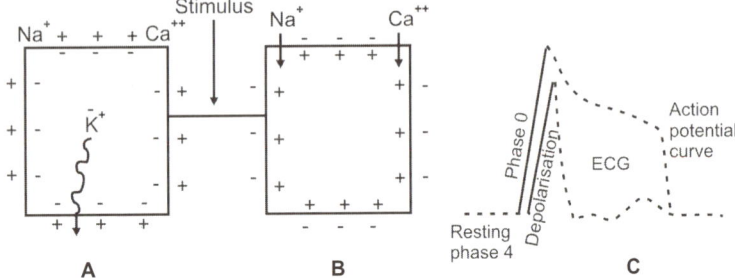

Figs 1.8A to C: Action potential. (A) Resting phase or polarised muscle cells; (B) Depolarised or stimulated muscle cell; (C) Resting action potential (phase 4) and action potential during activation (phase 0) on action potential curve that correlates with QRS on ECG

Repolarisation (Phases 1, 2 and 3)

Immediately after depolarisation (phase 0) of action potential, the muscle cell returns to its previous resting state through a process called *repolarisation,* which is recorded on the ECG as ST segment and T wave.

Phases 1, 2 and 3 of the action potential represent the repolarisation process (Fig. 1.9).

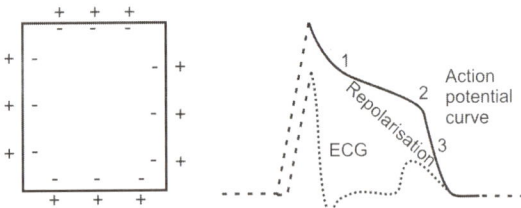

Fig. 1.9: Phases of repolarisation (1, 2, 3) with recovery of the cells. The inside of cell changes from positive back to its original resting negative charge. The phases (1, 2, 3) of repolarisation on action potential curve correlates with ST segment and T wave on ECG

What is the Shape of P-QRS-T Complex on ECG?

The shape of P-QRS-T complex recording the depolarisation and repolarisation of atria and ventricles is depicted in Fig. 1.10.

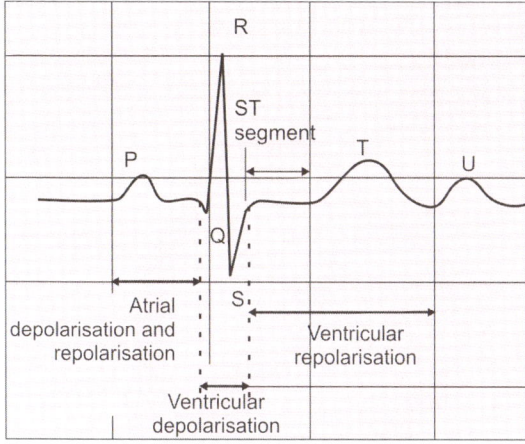

Fig. 1.10: The normal P-QRS-T complex

Waveforms of ECG (Box 1)

- *P wave:* An upward positive deflection that represents atrial depolarisation.
- *QRS complex:* It represents ventricular depolarisation.
- *T and U wave:* These waves represent ventricular repolarisation.

BOX 1: WAVEFORMS OF ECG
• First positive wave is called **P wave**
• First negative wave is called **Q wave**
• Second positive wave is large called **R wave**
• Second negative wave is small called **S wave**
• Third positive wave is called **T wave**
• Fourth positive wave if present is called **U wave**
Positive wave means deflection above the baseline and *negative* wave is deflection below the baseline.

The Genesis of P Wave

The SA node discharges spontaneously and regularly.

Genesis of P wave (atrial depolarization): It is due to automatic depolarisation and wave of excitation spreading to the atria and reaching the AV node via interconnecting pathways. When the atria are electrically activated, a P wave is recorded on the ECG (Fig. 1.11) which may be upright, inverted or biphasic in certain leads normally (Box 2).

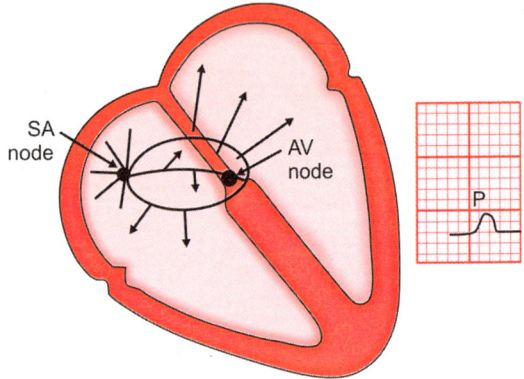

Fig. 1.11: Genesis of P wave (atrial depolarisation)

BOX 2: SHAPE OF P WAVE IN DIFFERENT LEADS
• Upright P: It is normally seen in leads I, II, aVF and V_3–V_6. • Upright or biphasic P wave in leads V_1–V_2 • Negative or inverted P wave in aVR • Depending on mean frontal axis, P wave may be upright or inverted in leads III and aVL.

The Genesis of QRS

i. *Genesis of normal Q wave:* It is produced due to septal activation from left to right normally (Fig. 1.12A). The Q wave will appear in the Q wave containing leads I, aVL and V_5–V_6.

Leads I, aVL, and V_5–V_6 are normal Q wave containing leads

ii. *Genesis of R wave:* After septal depolarisation, the wave of excitation spreads through the bundle branches to the ventricles and activates its free walls. The activation of right ventricle occurs ahead of left ventricle.

The left ventricle being dominant and having large muscle mass shifts the wave of excitation towards itself producing a

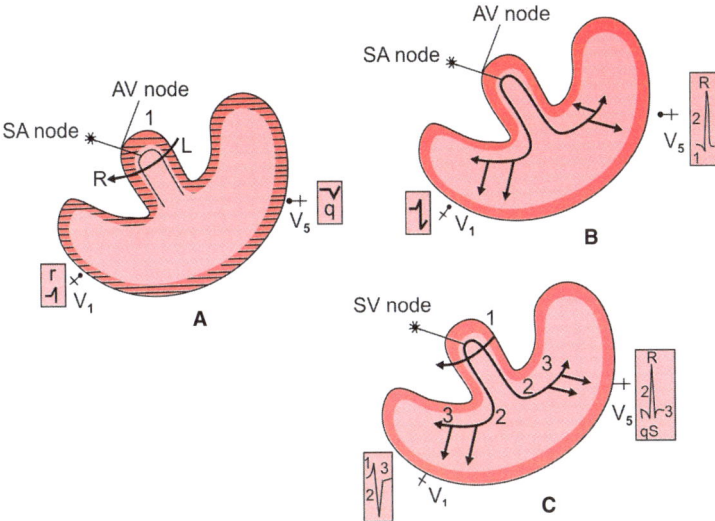

Figs 1.12A to C: Genesis of QRS. (A) Septal activation L → R (vector I) results in Q wave in left ventricular leads V_5–V_6 and R wave in right ventricular leads V_1–V_2; (B) Activation of dominant left ventricle shifts the activation front to the left (vector 2) resulting in R wave in V_5–V_6 and a corresponding S wave in V_1–V_2; (C) The activation of posterobasal segment (vector 3) results in S wave in V_5–V_6 but no wave is due to this activation in leads V_1–V_2

large R wave in left ventricular leads (V_5–V_6—Fig. 1.12B) and a corresponding S wave in right ventricular leads V_1–V_2 (wave of excitation is away from these leads); while the leads V_1–V_4 record both R and S, more or less of equal amplitude.

iii. *Genesis of S wave:* This is produced due to activation of posterobasal portion of the heart last of all. The S wave is seen in V_5–V_6 but no corresponding wave is seen in lead V_1–V_2 in majority of the cases (Fig. 1.12C).

iv. *Genesis of ST segment, T and U waves:* Ventricular depolarisation is followed by ventricular repolarisation which produces an isoelectric ST segment and an upright T wave, sometimes U wave also.

Ventricular repolarisation normally results in an isoelectric ST segment, upright T wave and U wave in all leads except aVR.

Nomenclature of QRS

Each lead has different shape of QRS complex. Each QRS complex is composed of multiple deflections above or below the baseline which are labelled as:

1. *The Q (q) wave:* First *downward deflection preceding an R wave*
2. *The R (r) wave:* First upward (positive) deflection.
3. *The S (s) wave:* The second downward or negative deflection that follows an R wave.
4. *The R' (r') wave:* Second positive deflection.

These waveforms have already been depicted (*Read* Box 1)

Note: A capital letter is used to denote a wave exceeding 5 mm; while a small letter is used if wave is less than 5 mm. The second upright R (r) wave is denoted as R' (r').

Based on the description of various deflections, the complexes encountered on ECG are given in Fig. 1.13.

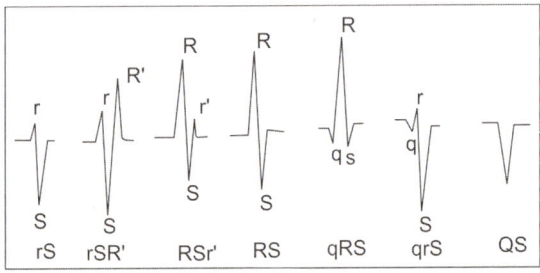

Fig. 1.13: QRS deflections and their nomenclature

Types of Ventricular Complexes (Figs 1.14A to C)

1. *Right ventricular epicardial complex:* It consists of a small r wave followed by a large S wave constituting rS complex. It is normally seen in leads representing the right ventricle on ECG, i.e. V_1 and V_2.
2. *Left ventricular epicardial complex:* It consists of a small q wave, a large R wave followed by an S wave constituting qRS complex. Sometimes, the terminal S is not recorded, hence, qR complex may just be seen. The normal qRS or qR

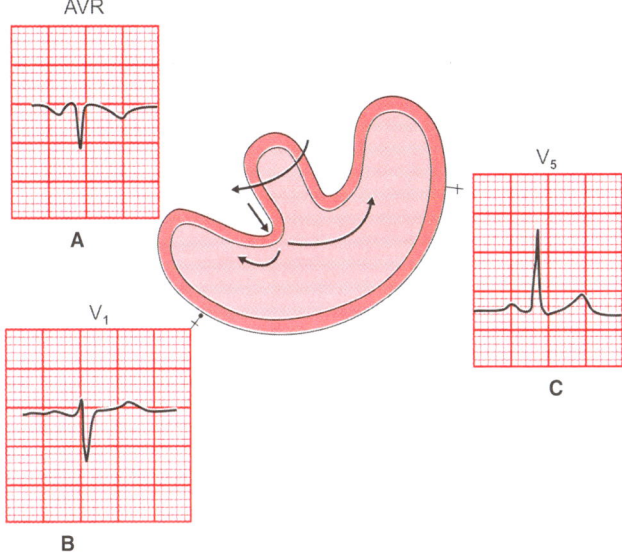

Figs 1.14A to C: Pathogenesis of various types of complexes. (A) Cavitary complex; (B) Right ventricular epicardial complex; (C) Left ventricular epicardial complex

complexes are seen in leads representing the left ventricle, i.e. leads V_1–V_6.

3. *Cavitary pattern:* It is a pattern consisting of all negative deflections, i.e. negative q wave, R wave and S wave. Normally, it is seen in lead aVR called cavitary lead.

The Physiology of R Wave Progression

The normal R wave progression means a gradual increase in the height of R wave in chest leads (V_1 to V_6) on ECG provided the chest leads have been placed at proper positions. This is due to the following reason:

The left ventricle is thicker (has 3 times more muscle mass) than right ventricles and lies to the left and behind right ventricle, hence, depolarisation of the left ventricle contributes to a large R wave in left precordial leads (V_5–V_6) as a result of which a large corresponding S is produced in leads V_1–V_2 and an equal R and S in leads V_3–V_4 (Figs 1.15A and B).

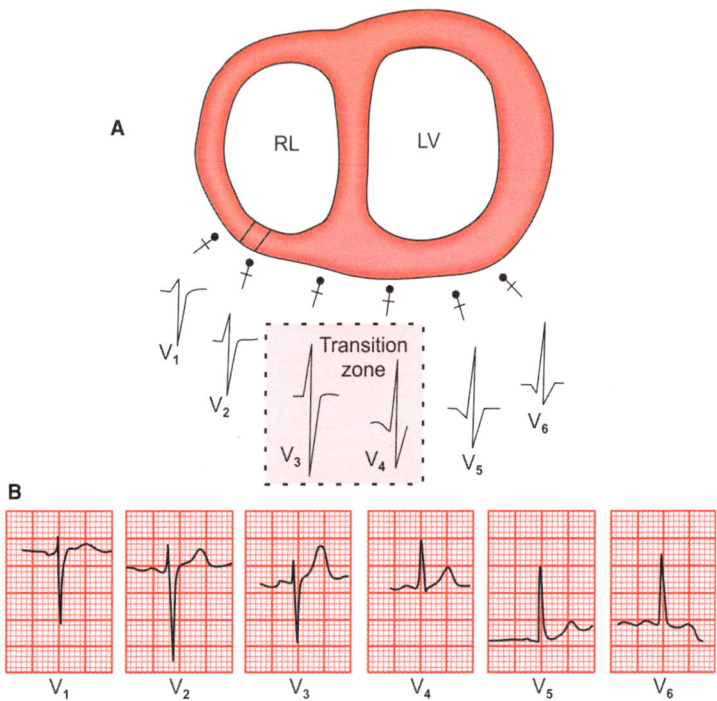

Figs 1.15A and B: (A) The R wave progression in precordial leads (diagram). Note R wave increase in height and S wave decreases as one proceeds from V₁ to V₆; (B) Normal R wave progression from V₁–V₆ on ECG

THE ELECTRICAL CARDIAC AXIS

What is Cardiac Axis?

Definition: The electrical cardiac axis means a net electrical force having direction and magnitude. An arrow (→) is used to indicate it because it has both direction and magnitude.

The Electrical Field of the Heart

The heart is situated in the centre of an electrical field. The intensity of the field decreases with the increase in the distance from the centre, thus, electrical intensity recorded by an electrode progressively diminishes as the electrode is progressively moved away from the heart. With distances greater than 15 cm away from the heart, the decrement in intensity of electrical field is minimally noticeable; which means that electrodes placed beyond 15 cm away from the heart, say 20, 30 and 40 cm away from the heart will record the same electrical potential. Using this principle, the electrodes are placed on the limbs away from the heart. These electrodes are considered to be equidistant from the heart.

Cardiac Vector and Shape of QRS

Now, we should know why does the ECG complex in each lead varies. This is due to direction of cardiac vector (Fig. 1.16).

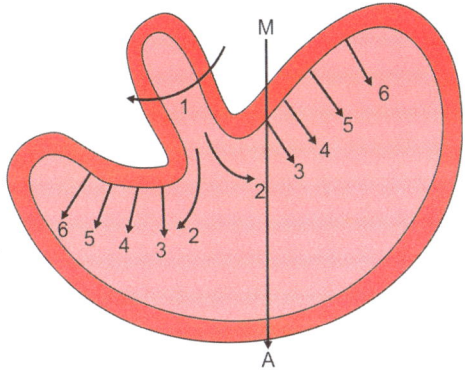

Fig. 1.16: Mean frontal plane axis (M→A). It is the mean of six instantaneous QRS vectors as shown

Depolarisation spreads through the heart in many directions at one time, but the shape of QRS shows the average or mean direction in which the wave of excitation is spreading through the heart called *cardiac vector*. The shape of the QRS depending on the direction of cardiac vector can be explained as follows:

1. If QRS is predominantly upward, or positive (i.e. R wave is greater than S wave), in a particular lead, the wave of excitation is moving towards the positive pole of that lead (Fig. 1.17A).

2. If QRS is predominantly downward or negative (S wave is greater than R wave), the wave of excitation is moving away from that lead (Fig. 1.17B).

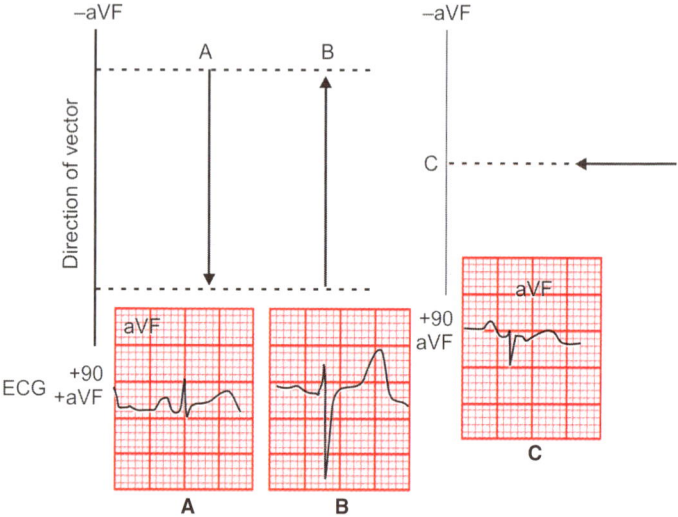

Figs 1.17A to C: Depolarisation (wave of excitation) and shape of the QRS. (A) Excitation wave is spreading towards the positive pole of lead aVF; (B) It is away from the lead, i.e. towards its negative pole; (C) It is perpendicular to that lead (aVF shown)

3. When wave of excitation is moving at right angle to that lead, the R and S waves are of equal magnitude and both are small (Fig. 1.17C) or may just have nil complex.

For example, sake, the effect of cardiac vector on leads I, II and III of ECG is depicted in Fig. 1.18.

The Hexaxial Reference System

The direction of ventricular depolarisation in each lead is called lead axis. The total QRS is determined by examining each of the *lead axes*. Also, each lead has a positive (+) and a negative (–) pole, and it is oriented in a certain direction in relation to heart.

The hexaxial references system places all the six standard leads (three bipolar and three unipolar) together into one picture so that a mean manifest QRS axis may be determined (Fig. 1.19). In this system, each lead is placed at an angle of 30° with respect to others.

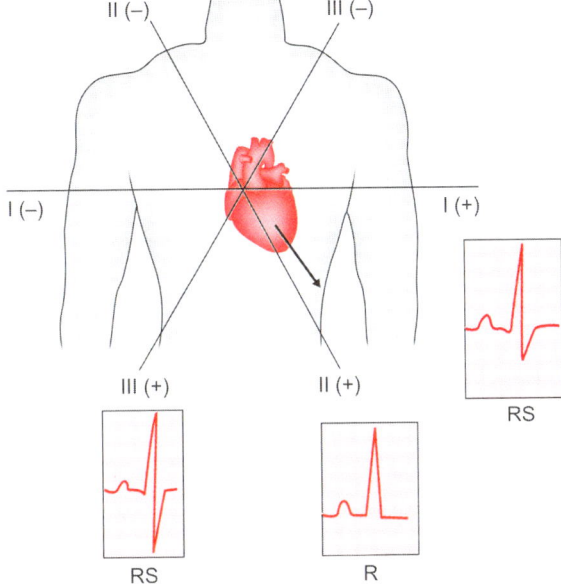

Fig. 1.18: The effect of QRS vector (mean indicated by an arrow →) on standard leads (I, II and III). The shape of QRS is different in each lead because each lead looks or faces depolarisation differently. The QRS vector is towards the positive pole of lead II, hence QRS has predominant upright R wave in that lead. The vector is oblique to lead I and III, hence there is large R wave and small S wave in these leads

How to Label the Hexaxial System?

By convention, all the degrees in the upper hemisphere of hexaxial system are labelled as negative (−) and in the lower hemisphere as positive (+). From the lead I (0°), progressing counterclockwise, the leads are labelled as −30°, −60°, −90°, +120°, −150° and −180; and progressing clockwise, from the same point, the successive leads are labelled as +30°, +60°, +90°, −120°, +150°, +180° (Fig. 1.19). The (+) and (−) degrees on the hexaxial system must not be confused with (+) and (−) poles of the lead axes. From the hexaxial reference system, it has become clear that (+) poles of standard leads (I, II, III, aVR, aVL and aVF) axes lie from −30° to +120° with an exception that negative pole of aVR is located at +30°.

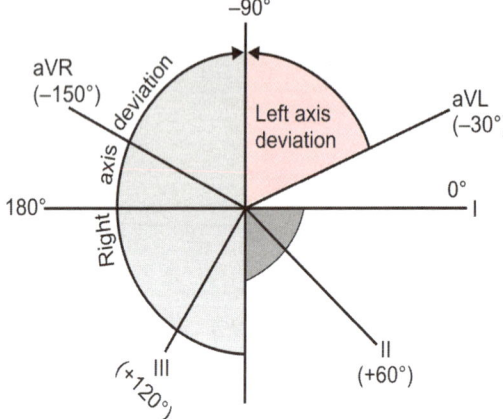

Fig. 1.19: The leads representation on hexaxial reference system and limits of normal and abnormal axes
- Normal axis extends from 0° to +90° is considered as normal.
- Right axis extends from +90° to –90°
- Left axis deviation extends from –30° to –90°.

Each lead axis in this system has a negative and a positive pole. It is useful to remember the location of positive pole of each lead on the hexaxial wheel. The positive pole of all standard leads except aVR lie in lower hemisphere; and negative poles in upper hemisphere except aVL.

> **Remember**
>
> *The positive pole of lead axes I, II and III are placed at 0°, +60° and +90° respectively (Fig. 1.19).*
>
> *The positive poles of lead axes aVR, aVL and aVF are placed at –150°, –30° and +90° respectively (Fig. 1.19).*

How to Determine QRS Axis?

The standard leads are used to calculate the axis.

> ***Rule 1:*** *When there is an equiphasic QRS (R = S) or a very small QRS or nil complex in any of the six leads and the mean QRS is perpendicular (⊥) to that lead.*

Examine all the six standard leads (I, II, III, aVR, aVL and aVF) carefully at a glance and find out.

Whether any lead has an equiphasic (R = S wave) complex or a very small or nil complex. If yes, e.g. in lead aVL (Fig. 1.20), then according to law of electrocardiography, the mean QRS axis is perpendicular to that lead whether positive or negative. Now, remember also that lead II is ⊥ to lead aVL (Fig. 1.19) hence, QRS axis is either towards the positive pole or negative pole of lead II. Now, examine lead II, if it has mainly positive deflection, then axis is +60° and if mainly negative then it is –60°.

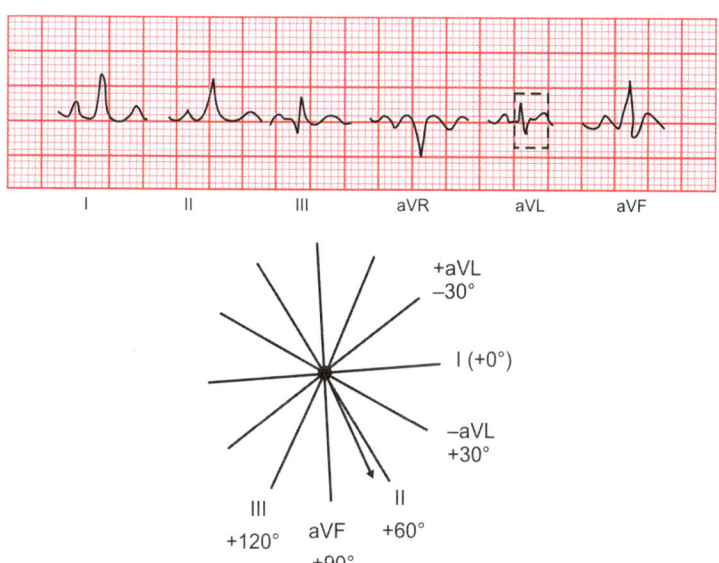

Fig. 1.20: The ECG shows a small equiphasic complex in aVL (squared). The QRS axis is perpendicular to aVL, i.e. towards lead II

Rule 2: *If two adjacent leads have either positive, or negative QRS deflection of equal size, then QRS axis lies midway between the two adjacent leads.*

Examine all the standard leads and find out any two adjacent standard leads having equal deflections either positive or negative, e.g. in Fig. 1.21, the leads II and aVF have equal positive deflection, hence, the QRS axis is midway between the two. The lead II on hexaxial system lies at +60° and aVF at

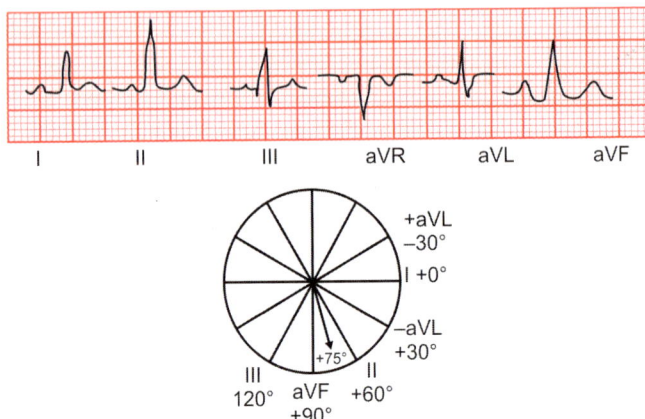

Fig. 1.21: In the ECG depicted, leads II and aVF have equal positive deflection, hence QRS axis is midway between the two, i.e. (60° + 90°) ÷ 2 = +75°

+90°, therefore, the QRS axis is (+60° +90°) ÷ 2 = + 75°. This method is called *bisector method.*

QUICK APPROXIMATION METHOD

This method determines axis by approximation

This gives an instantaneous rough estimate of abnormal axis deviation. In this method, two leads I and III are selected. Put the lead III below the lead I and calculate the approximate axis as demonstrated in Fig. 1.22.

The axis, i.e. normal and abnormal (right or left axis deviation) are represented below.

Put the QRS complex of lead III just below the lead I but not otherwise and then decide as follows:

1. *Right axis deviation:* The QRS deflections are right opposite to each other (Fig. 1.22A).

2. *Left axis deviation:* The QRS deflections are leaving apart each other (Fig. 1.22B).

3. *Normal axis:* The QRS deflections in both the leads are upright and they neither face each other nor drift away from each other (Fig. 1.22C).

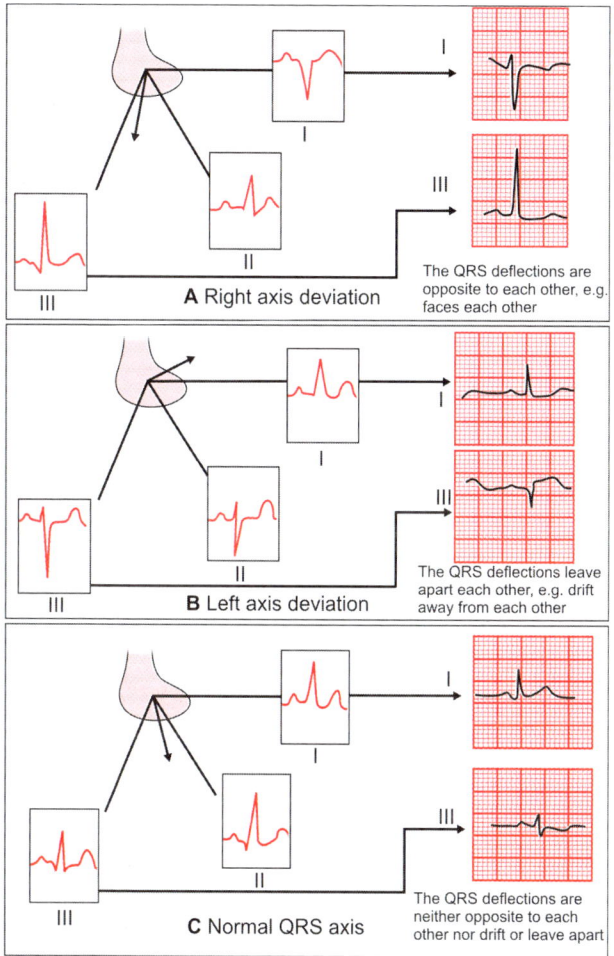

Figs 1.22A to C: The QRS axis calculation by approximation method (diagram)

Causes of Axis Deviation

They are given in Box 3.

THE ELECTRICAL ROTATION OF THE HEART

What does an Electrical Rotation Mean?

The electrical rotation of the heart means distribution and direction of electrical forces rather than shift in the anatomical

BOX 3: CAUSES OF AXIS DEVIATION

Right axis deviation
- Right ventricular hypertrophy
- Anterolateral MI
- Right bundle branch block
- Left posterior hemiblock

Left axis deviation
- Inferior wall infarction
- Left bundle branch block
- Left anterior hemiblock
- Left ventricular hypertrophy (LVH)
- Ventricular tachycardia with focus in left ventricle
- WPW syndrome.

position. Rotation here does not mean anatomical rotation but rotation or shift of electrical forces only.

Types

I. *Rotation around anteroposterior axis* (Fig. 1.23) which runs theoretically through the interventricular septum from anterior to posterior surface of the heart. This rotation occurs on frontal plane and is reflected in leads I, II, III, aVR, aVL and aVF. This type of rotation represents different heart positions as follows:

i. *Vertical heart position* (Figs 1.24A and B): In vertical heart position, the main body of left ventricle is oriented to leads II and aVF which records left ventricular epicardial complex (qR or qRS), and leads I and aVL record right ventricular (rS) complex.

ii. *Horizontal heart position* (Figs 1.25A and B): In this heart position, lead aVL faces left ventricle, hence, records qR or qRS complex and lead aVF faces right ventricle, hence records rS complex.

iii. *Intermediate heart position* (Figs 1.26A and B). This is midway position between vertical and horizontal heart positions. In this type, both the leads aVL and aVF record left ventricular epicardial complex (qR or qRS) Table 1.1.

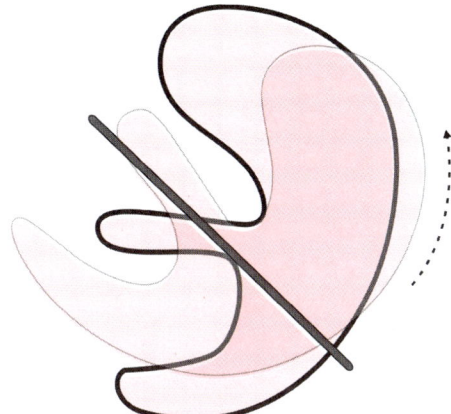

Fig. 1.23: Rotation around anteroposterior axis

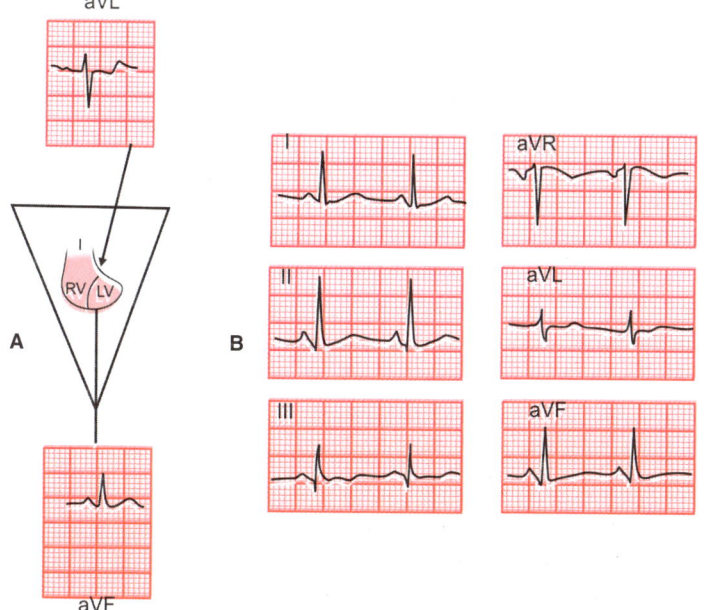

Figs 1.24A and B: Vertical heart position. (A) Diagram with recording of complexes. Only leads aVL and aVF displayed; (B) The ECG (standard 6 leads) shows aVL resembling normal V_1 (right ventricular epicardial complex), aVF resembling normal V_6 (left ventricular epicardial complexes) and aVR records inverted P and T with rS complex

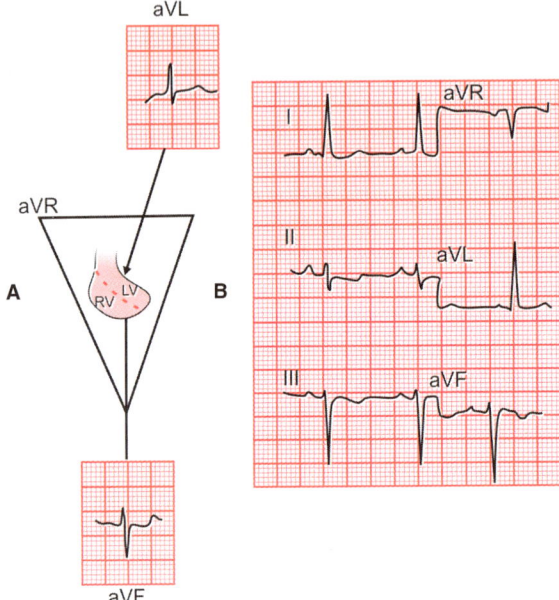

Figs 1.25A and B: Horizontal heart position. (A) Diagram; (B) The ECG shows left ventricular epicardial complex (qRS) in aVL resembling normal V_6 and right ventricular epicardial complex (rS) in aVF resembling normal V_1. Lead aVR records inverted P and T waves with rS complexes

Table 1.1: Heart positions on ECG		
Position	*Lead aVL*	*Lead aVF*
Vertical	rS	qR/qRS
Horizontal	qR/qRS	rS
Intermediate	qR/qRS	qR/qRS

II. *Rotation around horizontal or oblique axis* which runs through the interventricular septum from the apex to the base, is viewed from below the heart looking upwards towards the apex (Fig. 1.27). Rotation on this axis is called *clockwise* or *counterclockwise* is seen in the chest lead (V_1–V_6).

What does Transitional Zone Mean? What is its Significance?

Transitional zone or lead means an ECG complex which records an equiphasic R and S wave, i.e. R wave is equal to S wave.

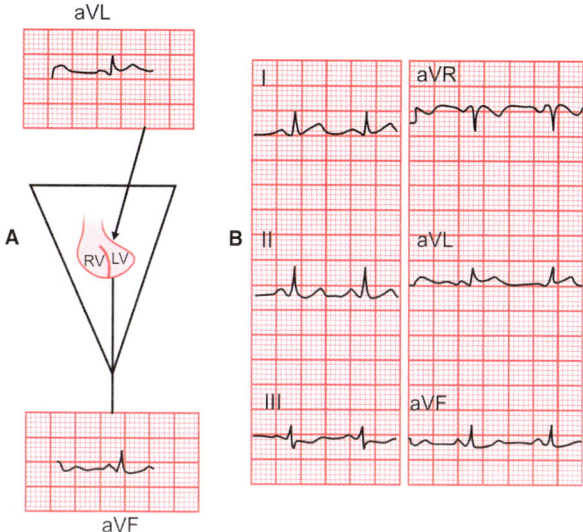

Figs 1.26A and B: Intermediate heart position. (A) Diagram with recording of ECG complex in aVL and aVF; (B) The ECG shows leads aVL and aVF resemble V_6, i.e. record left ventricular epicardial complex. The lead aVR shows inverted P and T waves and rSr' pattern

The zone or lead forms a transition between right ventricular and left ventricular complexes (*see* Fig. 1.15). It normally lies in leads V_3 or V_4 and indicate no rotation of heart.

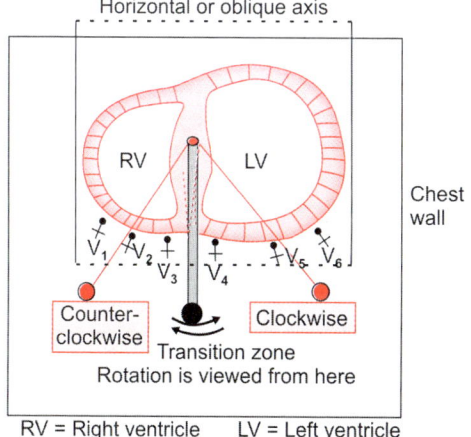

Fig. 1.27: Rotation around horizontal or oblique axis

The shift of this transition zone either clockwise (towards V_1 and V_2) or counterclockwise (towards V_5–V_6) indicate respective rotation (Figs 1.28A and B).

How to Determine Rotation?

Examine the chest leads (V_1–V_6) carefully at a glance. Note the progression of R wave and find out a chest lead having an equiphasic (R = S) complex. The lead having such a complex is called *transition lead* (*see* Fig. 1.15).

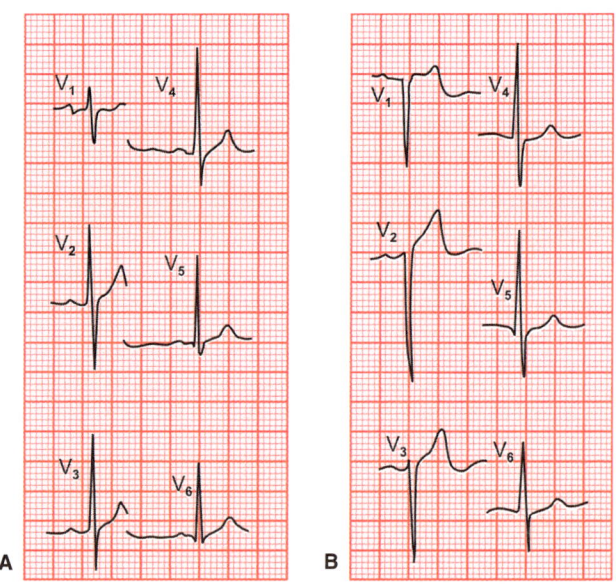

Figs 1.28A and B: The ECGs showing (A) Counterclockwise rotation (transition complex moves to V_2); (B) Clockwise rotation (transition complex moves to V_5 or V_6)

Now, note the shift of transition zone on ECG either to the left (reader's right) or to the right (reader's left). If transition zone (equiphasic complex R = S) is seen in V_5–V_6 instead of normal V_3 or V_4, it is called shift to the left or *clockwise rotation*; if it is seen in lead V_1 or V_2, it is called *counterclockwise rotation* or shift to the right (Figs 1.28A and B). If the transition zone lies normally, it is called no shift.

2

Normal Electrocardiogram

- Normal ECG recording
- Components of an ECG complex
  - Waveforms, e.g. P, Q, R, S, T and U waves
  - Intervals, e.g. P-R, R-R, Q-T/QTc
  - Segment, e.g. ST

What is the Electrocardiographic Paper?

The electrocardiographic (ECG) paper is a graph paper with horizontal and vertical lines at 1 mm distance that intersect to form small and large squares respectively. Vertical measurement reflects voltage and horizontal measurement reflects time. Each small square is equal to 1 mm; 0.04 sec in time and 0.1 mV in height. Each large square is bounded by a heavier or dark line, consists of 5 small squares (5 mm), reflects 0.5 mV (height) and 0.2 second in duration (Fig. 2.1). After every five big square, the darker line extends onto the white upper border of ECG paper.

How would you Calculate Heart Rate?

1. *If heart rate is regular* then heart rate is calculated by R-R method.

   The R-R method (Fig. 2.2): Divide 1500 by number of small squares counted in-between two consecutive QRS complexes to get the heart rate. For example, if there are 20 small squares in-between two successive R-R complexes, then heart rate is $1500 \div 20 = 75/\text{min}$.

2. *If rhythm is irregular*, then heart rate is calculated by six second method:

   i. *Six second method* (Fig. 2.3): Count the number of QRS within 6 seconds (within 30 big squares or within 6 dark

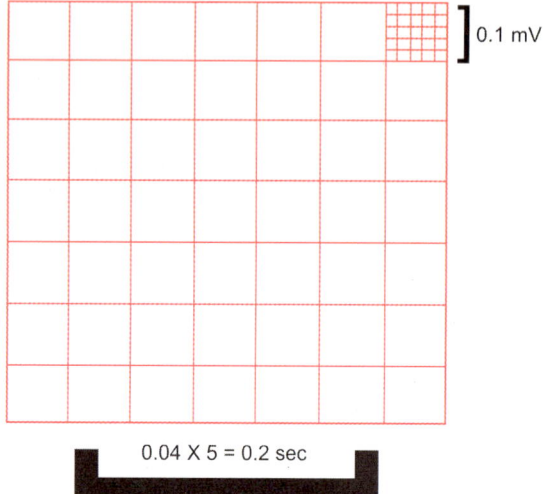

Fig. 2.1: The ECG paper

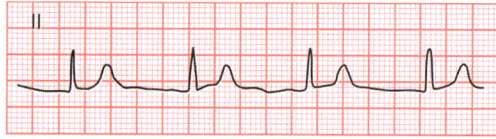

Fig. 2.2: Calculation of heart rate by R-R method. The R-R interval is 23 small squares, HR = 1500 ÷ R-R = 1500 ÷ 23 = 65/min

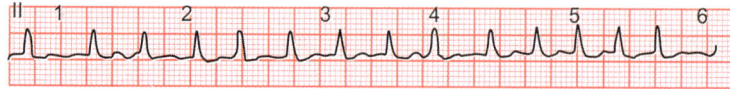

Fig. 2.3: Calculation of heart rate by 6 sec method. The basic rhythm is irregular due to atrial fibrillation. There are 13 QRS complexes within 6 seconds. The heart rate is 13 × 10 = 130/min (approx)

lines representing the time marker) and multiply the number obtained by 10 to get the approximate heart rate in one minute. This method is used in patients of atrial fibrillation to know the ventricular rate.

Voltage Measurement

It is an essential parameter for electrocardiographic interpretation. The voltage of an upright deflection is measured from the baseline to the top of deflection. The voltage of a negative deflection is measured from lower portion of the baseline to the bottom of the wave (Fig. 2.4). The voltage of QRS includes both positive and negative deflections.

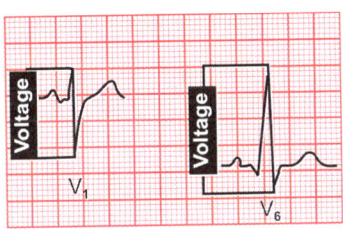

Fig. 2.4: The voltage measurement

Low voltage graph (Fig. 2.5). If the voltage of QRS does not exceed 5 mm in standard leads (I, II, III, aVR, aVL and aVF) and / or 10 mm in the precordial leads (V_1 to V_6), then, it is called a *low voltage graph*. The conditions associated with low voltage graph are given in Box 1.

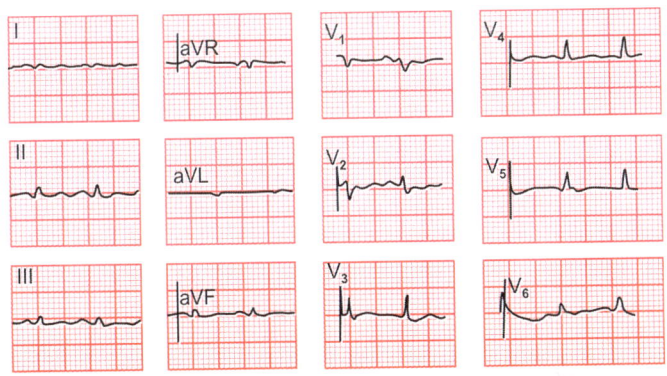

Fig. 2.5: Low voltage graph. Note no QRS complex exceeds 5 mm in standard leads (I, II, III, aVR, aVL and aVF) and 10 mm in precordial leads (V_1–V_6)

The high voltage of QRS complexes is seen in ventricular hypertrophy (read ventricular hypertrophy).

NORMAL ELECTROCARDIOGRAM

To define normalcy in electrocardiography is not only difficult but impossible task because of so many normal variations and

BOX 1: CAUSES OF LOW VOLTAGE GRAPH	
• COPD mainly emphysema	• Massive bilateral or left-sided pleural effusion
• Myxoedema	• Obesity (extreme)
• Pericardial effusion or cardiac tamponade	• Left pneumothorax
• Grossly dilated heart such as in dilated cardiomyopathy	• Oedematous chest wall (anasarca)

physiological conditions affecting the ECG. Conventionally, it is better to say that electrocardiogram is within normal limits rather than a normal electrocardiogram.

The normal electrocardiogram means normal heart rate (60–100 bpm), sinus rhythm, normal QRS axis and a normal P-QRS-T complex (Fig. 2.6) provided the electrodes placement and ECG recording has been done under proper conditions.

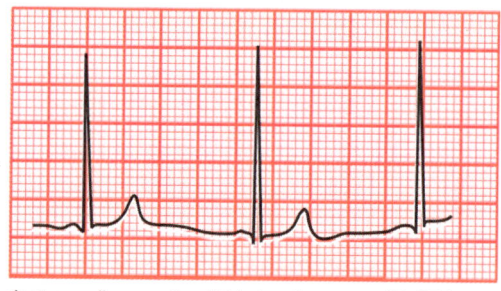

Fig. 2.6: The electrocardiogram (lead V_5) showing normal P-QRS-TU characteristics

COMPONENTS OF AN ECG COMPLEX

Normally, an ECG complex (Fig. 2.7) consists of:
1. *Waveforms:* P-QRS-TU
2. *Segments:* PR and ST
3. *Junction:* QRS-T junction called J point
4. *Intervals:* P-P, R-R, P-R, QRS and Q-T (QTc)

The Normal P Wave (Fig. 2.8)

It is produced by atrial depolarisation, best seen in leads I, II, III and aVF. It is usually upright in all leads except aVR where

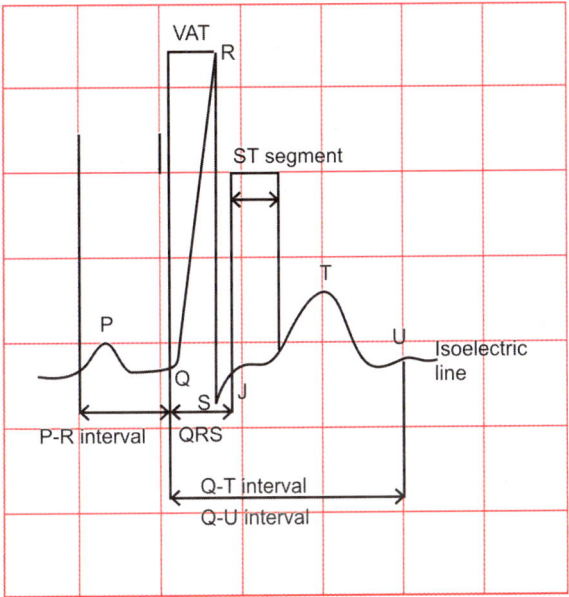

Fig. 2.7: Normal electrocardiogram showing waveforms, segments, junctions and intervals

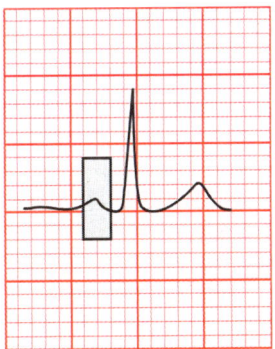

Fig. 2.8: The P wave in frontal plane leads (shaded)

it is always inverted. It can be inverted in leads III and aVL. P wave may be normally biphasic, i.e. have both upward or positive and downward or negative reflection) in lead V_1 and sometimes in V_2. The P wave characteristic are given in Box 2.

- Shape – upright
- Height ≤ 2.5 mm
- Duration 0.08 to 0.10 sec but not > 0.11 sec in any circumstance
- Visibility – best seen in leads I, II and aVF because P wave axis lies between +40° and +60°

The Normal QRS (Fig. 2.9)

It is produced by ventricular depolarisation, is positive in all leads except aVR and is equiphasic (R = S) in leads V_3 and V_4.

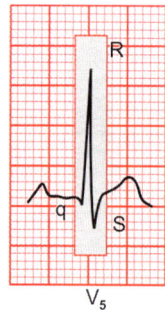

Fig. 2.9: A normal QRS in lead V_5 (shaded)

The Q (q) Wave

The Q wave is seen normally in q wave containing leads, i.e. I, aVL, V_5 and V_6. It is less than 0.04 sec (less than one small square) in width and depth, beyond which it is considered as abnormal, i.e. an abnormal q wave is > 0.04 both in height and width; is seen in acute myocardial infarction and hypertrophic cardiomyopathy (septal hypertrophy). The q wave is lost in left bundle branch block.

Remember

The q wave precedes R wave in QRS complex, is negative wave of < 0.04 sec of width and depth.

The R Wave

The R wave in QRS complex is first positive wave and does not exceed 25 mm in height in any lead. Its amplitude increases in ventricular hypertrophy. Its amplitude progressively increases from V_1–V_6 so that it is tallest in V_5 a phenomenon called *normal* R *wave progression*.

The characteristics and morphology of QRS are depicted in Fig. 2.9.

Characteristics of QRS Complex

- Width or duration of QRS is 0.04 to 0.10 sec, but should not exceed 0.11 sec in any lead normally.
- The VAT (ventricular activation time) is measured from the beginning of q wave to top of the R wave, is 0.03 sec in right oriented leads (V_1–V_2) and 0.05 sec in left oriented leads (V_5–V_6).
- A transition complex consisting of an R and a S wave of equal amplitude, is normally seen in V_3 or V_4.

The S Wave

The S wave is second negative deflection in QRS complex, produced by depolarisation of basal portion of the heart. Normally, as R wave progresses in height from V_1 to V_6, the S wave decreases in depth from V_1 to V_6, hence, it is smallest in V_6.

The QRS deflection and nomenclature: It has already been discussed in the previous section.

The Normal T Wave (Fig. 2.10)

The normal T wave is a positive deflection representing the ventricular repolarization. The T wave amplitude diminishes with age. It is taller in athletes: It is normally upright in all leads except aVR where it is inverted. Normally, it does not exceed 30–35% of the R wave in chest leads but if it is 75% of R wave in chest leads, it is called tall T wave. Tall or relatively tall T waves are frequently seen normally in mid-precordial leads. The characteristics of normal T wave are given in Box 3.

The T wave is normally inverted in leads V_1 to V_3 in infants and children due to normal right ventricular dominance. This pattern of T wave inversion, occasionally, persists in adults called *persistent juvenile pattern*.

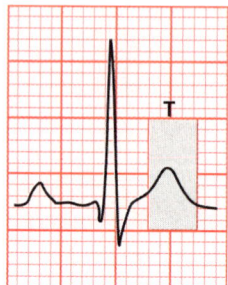

Fig. 2.10: Normal T wave (shaded)

BOX 3: CHARACTERISTICS OF NORMAL T WAVE
• It is an upright deflection in all leads except aVR
• It has a blunt apex and follows QRS complex after ST segment
• It is inscribed in the same direction as QRS complex

The U Wave

The normal U wave is small, shallow, rounded upward deflection inscribed after the T wave. It indicates delayed ventricular repolarisation. Normally, it is best seen in leads V_3–V_4. It is 1 mm in amplitude, is prominent in athletes. It becomes prominent in certain conditions such as hypokalaemia. It may become inverted in myocardial ischaemia infarction.

The Normal ECG Intervals

1. *The P-R interval:* It is measured from the beginning of P wave to the beginning of Q wave of QRS complex or R wave of QRS, if Q wave is not seen. It actually represents the time taken by the sinus impulse to reach the ventricle through atria and AV node. The normal P-R is 0.12 to 0.20 sec interval at normal heart rate. It is diagrammatically illustrated in Fig. 2.11.

2. *The QRS interval* (Fig. 2.12): It is measured from the beginning of QRS to its end point called 'J' point. It actually represents the time taken by the impulse to depolarise the septum and ventricles from endocardial to epicardial surface. The characteristics of QRS complex has already been discussed.

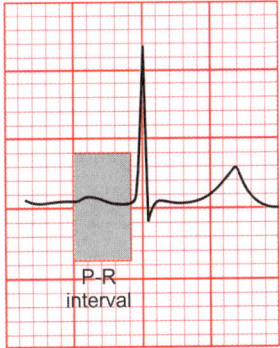

Fig. 2.11: Normal P-R interval (shaded)

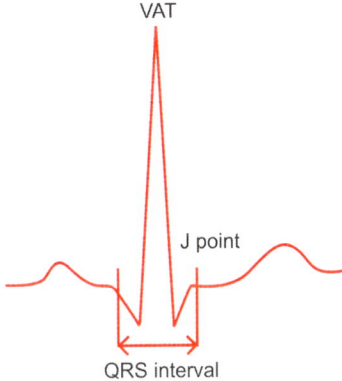

Fig. 2.12: The QRS interval (diag)

Ventricular activation time (VAT) represents the beginning to the peak of ventricular depolarisation, is measured from the beginning of Q wave to the top of R wave (Fig. 2.13).

The Q-T Interval (Fig. 2.14)

The interval between the beginning of QRS to the end of T wave is called *Q-T interval*. It represents the total activation of ventricles (depolarisation cum repolarisation). It varies with heart rate for which it is corrected called corrected QT (QTc) interval and is calculated as follows:

$$\text{QTc (Bazett's formula)} = \frac{Q\text{-}T \ interval \ in \ sec}{\sqrt{R\text{-}R}}$$

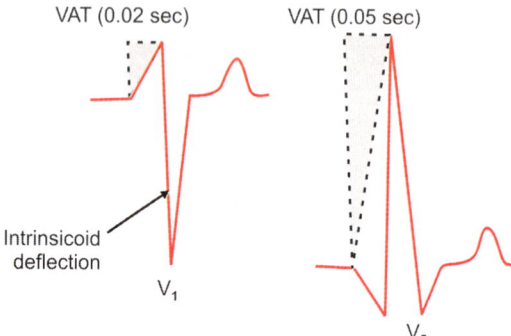

Fig. 2.13: Normal ventricular activation time in right (V_1) and left (V_5) precordial leads

The characteristics of Q-T (QTc) along with morphology of Q-T is represented in the (Fig. 2.14).

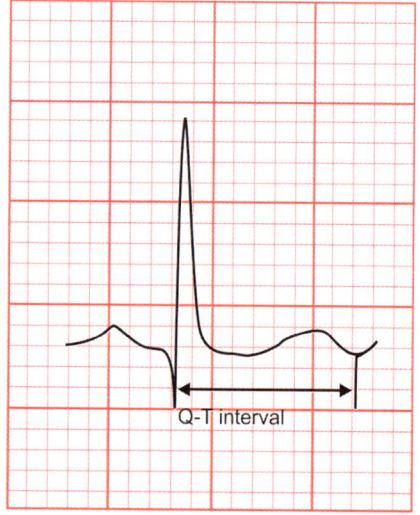

Fig. 2.14: The Q-T interval

- It varies with age, sex and heart rate. It is longer in female, in old age and during slow heart rate.
- *Normal QTc:* It is < 0.40 sec in males and < 0.45 sec in females (0.39 ± 0.04 sec).

Abnormalities of QTc occur in the form of prolongation and shortening (Figs 2.15A to C) the causes of which are given in Box 4.

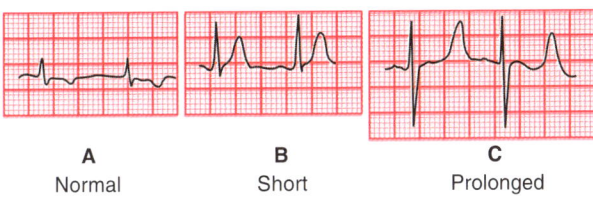

A	B	C
Normal	Short	Prolonged

Figs 2.15A to C: Long and short QTc

BOX 4: CAUSES OF LONG AND SHORT QT (QTc)	
Long QTc	*Short QTc*
1. Congenital	• Digitalis effect
• Physiological during sleep	• Hyperthermia
• Congenital prolonged QT syndrome, e.g. the Jervell and Lange-Nielsen syndrome and Romano-Ward syndrome	• Vagal stimulation
2. Acquired	
• Hypocalcaemia	
• Myocarditis	
• Acute myocardial infarction	
• Quinine, Quinidine, procainamide and tricyclic or tetracyclic antidepressants	
• Head injury or CVA	
• Hypothermia	

The P-P Interval (Fig. 2.16)

It is the interval between two successive P waves. It is measured from the beginning of first P wave to the beginning of next P wave. It is used to calculate atrial rate similar to R-R method used to calculate ventricular rate, i.e. 1500 ÷ R-R or P-P interval provided heart rate is regular. The clinical importance lies when atrial rate is different than ventricular rates, e.g. in AV dissociation and complete heart block.

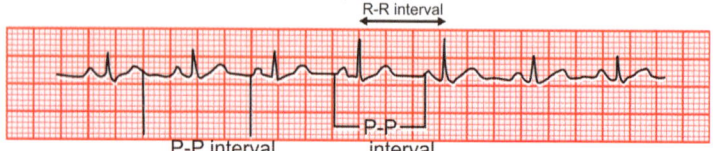

Fig. 2.16: Normal P-P and R-R intervals. Atrial rate (P-P interval) and ventricular rate (R-R interval) is 87/min

The R-R Interval (Fig. 2.16)

It is measured between two successive R waves, i.e. measured from the beginning of one R wave to the beginning of next R wave. The R-R interval is regular like P-P interval in sinus rhythm. It is used to calculate ventricular rate. Slight variation in R-R interval may occur due to respiratory effect called *respiratory sinus arrhythmia*. Irregular R-R intervals indicate disturbance in atrial, nodal and ventricular rhythm.

Normal Segments and Junctions

1. *PR Segment* (Fig. 2.17)

It is the distance between the end of the P wave to the beginning of QRS complex. Normally, it is isoelectric, hence, is used as baseline to evaluate the deviation of ST segment.

2. *The ST Segment*

It is the distance from the end of S wave to the beginning of T wave. The point at which the S wave joins the baseline is called *J point*. Therefore, actually the distance from the J point to the onset of T wave is ST segment and is usually isoelectric. The ST segment merges with T wave.

Deviation of ST segment (elevation or depression) is decided with reference to an isoelectric TP line or segment (Fig. 2.17). The causes of ST segment elevation and depression have been discussed in Chapter 5.

3. *The TP Segment*

It is the portion of tracing between the end of T wave and the beginning of the next P wave. It is an isoelectric segment used as reference (baseline) to determine the deviation of ST segment from the baseline.

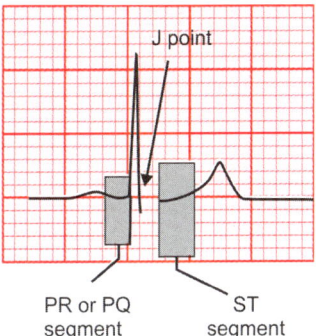

Fig. 2.17: The normal PQ and ST segments (shaded)

4. The R-S Junction (J point)

The R-S junction is called *'J' point* at which QRS ends with S wave returning to the baseline and ST segment starts. The 'J' point in electrocardiography (resting or stress) is important for evaluation of initial ST segment deviation, i.e. elevation/depression (Fig. 2.17).

NORMAL ELECTROCARDIOGRAM IN ADULTS (Fig. 2.18)

The electrocardiogram is interpreted with reference to the followings:
1. *Standardisation:* Normal (10 mm or 1 mV)
2. Rate (60–100 bpm)
3. *Voltage:* It should not be low voltage. The normal voltage is not defined.
4. *Axis:* Mean frontal plane QRS is 0° to +90°.
5. *Position:* The normal heart has an intermediate position
6. *Rotation:* Normally, there is no rotation, i.e. transition zone lies either in V_3 or V_4 or in-between the two.
7. *The P wave:* The normal P does not exceed 2.5 mm in width or height.
8. *The P-R interval:* It is 0.12 to 0.20 sec at normal heart rate and 0.22 sec at heart rate of 60/min is taken as upper limit of normal.
9. *QRS complex:* In standard leads, there is dominant R wave. In V_1 the normal pattern is rS. Gradually, the height of R wave increases and S wave decreases from V_1–V_6.

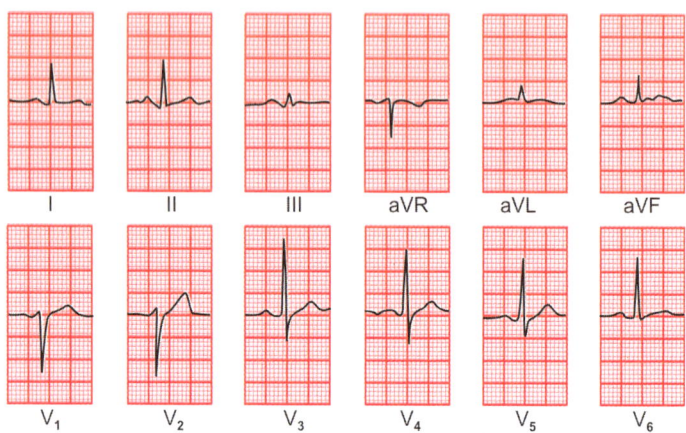

Fig. 2.18: Normal ECG showing normal P wave, P-R interval, normal QRS, normal ST segment and T wave

10. *QRS duration:* It is from 0.04 to 0.10 sec.
11. *The ST segment:* The normal ST segment is isoelectric.
12. *The T wave:* The T wave is normally inscribed in the same direction as the QRS complex. It is usually upright except in leads aVR and V_1.
13. *QT (QTc) interval:* The normal QTc interval is < 0.40 sec in males and < 0.45 sec in females.
14. *The U wave:* Normally, the U wave is not seen, if seen, it is best in amplitude in leads V_3–V_4. Its amplitude is less than T wave.

The ECG must be interpreted under the heads described above. The abnormal findings must be highlighted. No diagnosis should be made on ECG findings. Conclusion drawn should be written that findings are suggestive of.............. or the findings should be co-related with the clinical findings.

3

Conduction Disturbance

- Conduction disturbance through AV node, i.e. heart or AV blocks
- Conduction disturbance through bundle branches, i.e. bundle branch blocks
- Conduction disturbance through the fascicles of left bundle branch, i.e. fascicular block
- Bifascicular blocks
- Accelerated conduction, i.e. WPW syndrome

HEART OR ATRIOVENTRICULAR (AV) BLOCKS

As already discussed, the sinus impulse travels to AV node through atria. In AV node, the impulse is slightly delayed called *physiological delay*. From AV node, it spreads to ventricles via bundle of His and bundle branches.

The conduction of the wavefront or the impulse can be delayed or blocked at any point.

What does AV Block Mean?

The delay or block of the impulse in AV node is called *heart block/AV block*.

Types

- First degree AV block
- Second degree AV block
- Complete AV block

First Degree AV Block

First degree AV block occurs due to delayed conduction between the SA node and the ventricles. The P-R interval normally represents time taken by the sinus impulse to reach the ventricles hence, consists of time taken from SA node to

AV node *plus* physiological delay in AV node *plus* impulse conduction from AV node to the ventricles. In first degree AV block, P-R interval is prolonged and underlying rhythm is preserved.

Remember

Normally, there is slight delay of sinus impulses in AV node: Further delay results in first degree AV block.

Causes

1. Vagotonaemia
2. Acute rheumatic carditis
3. Drugs, e.g. digoxin, betablcokers and calcium channel blockers
4. Coronary artery disease (e.g. inferior wall infarction)
5. Congenital heart disease (e.g. ASD and Ebstein's anomaly)
6. Myocarditis
7. Degeneration of conducting pathways associated with ageing.
8. Idiopathic

The ECG characteristic (Fig. 3.1)

1. The rhythm is regular (P-P and R-R intervals are constant).
2. Each P is followed by QRS, hence, there is no dropped beat.
3. The P-R interval is consistently prolonged beyond 0.20 sec at normal heart rate and 0.22 sec at a heart rate of 60/min.
4. The QRS complex is narrow and normal.

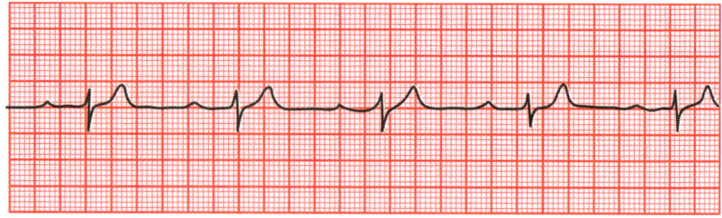

Fig. 3.1: First degree AV block. The P-R interval is 0.32 sec

Second Degree AV Block

In this type of block, there is intermittent failure or interruption of AV conduction with the result some of the sinus impulses are conducted to the ventricles while others are blocked producing a pause. The P wave formation is normal.

Causes

1. Physiological—athletes, vagotonic individual.
2. Acute rheumatic carditis.
3. Myocardial infarction (e.g. inferior wall and right ventricular).
4. Acute diphtheric myocarditis.
5. Drugs—digitalis toxicity.
6. Aortic valve disease (aortitis).
7. Infiltrative heart disease, e.g. amyloidosis.
8. Idiopathic fibrosis of conduction system (Lenegre's disease).
9. Calcification of mitral or aortic or both valve.

Remember

In second degree AV block, one or more P waves are absent intermittently in the rhythm strip.

In second degree AV block, there is intermittent dropping of a beat or beats in a sequence called *conduction ratio*. Conduction ratio is defined as ratio of number of P waves to number of QRS complexes in one sequence; the sequence begins with first conducted P wave after the pause, and ends with the next dropped P wave and includes this P wave in the sequence. For examiple, suppose there are four P waves in one sequence; but QRS complexes are three indicating only 3 P have been conducted then the conduction ratio is 4:3. Thus, one can label second degree AV block as 2:1, 3:2, 4:3, 5:4, 6:5, etc.

Types

Mobitz type I (Wenckebach) AV block

It is characterized by progressive lengthening of successive P-R intervals till one P is blocked (i.e. not followed by QRS) creating a pause on ECG. This pause due to dropped beat allows the conduction system to recover.

In Mobitz type I (Wenckebach) block, the QRS complexes appear in clusters, in a cycle called **group beating**. The period of a group beating is called **Wenckebach period**.

The ECG characteristics of Mobitz type I (Wenckebach) block (Fig. 3.2)

1. The basic rhythm is sinus. The P-P intervals are constant. The QRS complexes are narrow.

2. The P-R interval of successive heats progressively lengthen in a cyclic manner (group beating is present) until one P is blocked (not followed by QRS) following which cycle repeats again.

3. The R-R intervals are irregular due to dropped beats causing QRS complexes to appear in groups called *group beating*.

4. The conduction ratio varies, e.g. 4:3, 5.4, 6:5 or greater.

☞ **Clinical clue:** *In Mobitz type I (Wenckebach) AV block, there is progressive lengthening of successive P-R intervals till one P is blocked, i.e. pause appears.*

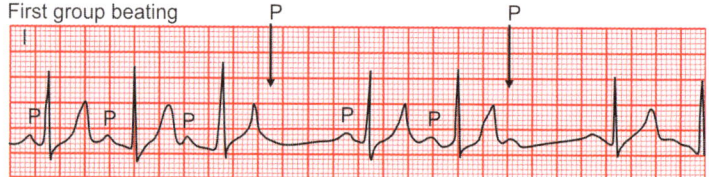

Fig. 3.2: Second degree Mobitz type I AV block (Wenckebach's block). There are group beatings. First group consists of 4 P waves in which 3 are conducted and 4th is blocked (↓) indicating 4:3 AV block. There is progressive lengthening of P-R intervals of first 3 P waves and the 4th P is blocked indicating Wenckebach type of conduction. In second group, out of 3 P waves 2 are conducted (3:2 block)

Mobitz type II AV block

In this type of block, the P-R interval of all conducted beats remains constant but there is intermittent dropping of beats (some P waves are not followed by QRS) There is no **Wenckebach's phenomenon.**

The ECG characteristics (Fig. 3.3)

1. P-R interval of the conducted beats is constant and fixed.

2. P-P intervals are constant and regular at a rate of 84/min.

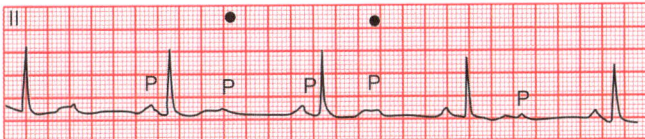

Fig. 3.3: Second degree Mobitz type II AV block. The lead II shows fixed P-R interval of 0.14 sec; one P wave is conducted while other is blocked (●) indicating 2:1 Mobitz II AV block. The atrial rate is 88/min and ventricular rate is 42/min

3. The R-R interval is regular or variable intermittently due to dropping of beats producing pauses.
4. The conduction ratio may be fixed (3:1, 2:1) or variable.

☛ *In Mobitz type II block, certain sinus beats are conducted and some are blocked in a variable or fixed fashion.*

Complete (Third Degree) AV Block

This is characterised by complete interruption of AV conduction between atria and ventricles, i.e. the supraventricular or sinus beats are blocked within the AV node. Therefore, to maintain the cardiac rhythm, there are two independent pacemakers; one in the SA node or in atrium and the other lies below the level of obstruction in the AV node (e.g. bundle of His, a bundle branch or a ventricle). These two pacemakers beat independently and asynchronously producing two rhythms (atrial and ventricular) which are not related. The ventricular rhythm is called *idioventricular rhythm*.

Remember

In complete heart block, no supraventricular beat is conducted to the ventricles due to complete barricade at the level of AV node. There is an idioventricular rhythm.

Causes

1. Drugs, e.g. digoxin, beta blockers and calcium channel blockers.
2. Hypervagotonaemia.
3. Acute MI (inferior wall or right ventricular infarction). In MI, the complete heart block is transient and may require placement of pacemaker.

4. Congenital AV block.
5. Acute rheumatic carditis.
6. Congenital heart disease (ostium primum ASD, VSD, etc.).
7. Lenegre's idiopathic degeneration and fibrosis of conduction system.
8. Lev's disease (fibrocalcareous encroachment).
9. Myocarditis, pericarditis, Chagas's disease is the commonest cause of AV block is central and South America.
10. Intracardiac surgery.
11. Amyloid heart disease, myxomatous infiltration, etc.
12. Space occupying lesions close to AV node (e.g. tuberculoma, gumma and tumour).

The ECG characteristic (Figs 3.4 and 3.5)

1. The P-P and R-R intervals are constant.
2. The atrial and ventricular rates are different. The atrial rate is faster than ventricular. The ventricular rate depends on the origin of subsidiary pacemaker, hence, varies from 15–60/min but usually lies between 15 and 45/min.
3. There is no relationship between P waves and QRS complexes, i.e. there is complete dissociation between P waves and QRS complexes.
4. QRS complexes are wider than normal.
5. The basic rhythm is either sinus or one of supraventricular type (e.g. atrial tachycardia, atrial flutter, atrial fibrillation, etc.).

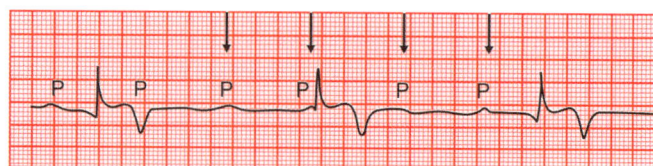

Fig. 3.4: Complete heart block. The P waves are nicely seen, (↓) P-P interval is regular. The QRS is wide and bizarre. The P-R interval is variable indicating P wave has no fixed relation to QRS. The heart rate is just 30/min indicating an idioventricular rhythm. The QRS complexes have a q wave, slightly elevated ST segment and symmetrically inverted T waves indicating the cause of complete heart block as ischaemia/infarction

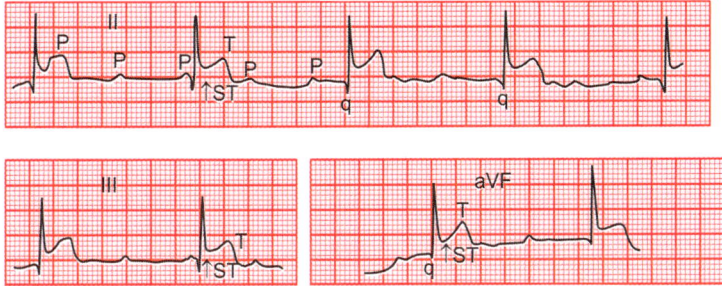

Fig. 3.5: Complete heart block (third degree) in a patient with inferior wall infarction. (i) *Evidence of complete heart block.* The lead II shows constant and fixed P-P and R-R intervals with no relation of P wave with QRS. The QRS is wider than normal; (ii) *Evidence of inferior wall infarction.* The ECG leads II, III and aVF show Q waves and elevated ST segment with dragged up T waves

> *Remember*
>
> *In atrial fibrillation the regular R-R intervals indicate associated complete heart block.*

How to Diagnose AV Block on ECG?

> *Remember*
>
> *A single strip is sufficient for this purpose.*

1. Look at the R-R interval. Is it regular or irregular?
2. Look at P waves. Is there only one P or more than one P for every QRS?
3. Look at the P-R interval. Is it same or does it change?

Analysis

I. **When R-R interval is regular** and the block is likely to be either first degree or third degree (complete) AV block.

- If P-R interval stays the same and each P wave is followed by a QRS complex after an interval of > 0.20 sec, it is first degree AV block.
- If P-R interval is variable and there is more than one P for every QRS, and both P wave and QRS do not maintain constant relationship and are independent, then it is complete AV block.

II. **If R-R interval is irregular**, the block is likely to be second degree because P waves are intermittently blocked.

- If P-R interval changes, i.e. lengthens with each successive beat till one P is dropped, then it is Mobitz type I (Wenckebach) AV block.
- If P-R interval is fixed, then it is Mobitz type II AV block.

Clinical significance

The second degree AV block may change to third degree AV block, and in transition, may produce **Stokes-Adams attacks** (syncopal attack during supine position). They are seen in complete heart block but are infrequent per se.

NB: The complete heart block is an indication of pacemaker insertion.

BUNDLE BRANCH BLOCKS (BBBs)

Since conduction from SA node to AV node is normal in bundle branch block, hence, P wave and P-R interval are normal. However, if conduction is delayed either through the right or left bundle branch (bundle branch block) then there will be delay in the depolarisation of the part of ventricle activated by that bundle branch. Therefore, an extra time will be taken for depolarisation of the whole of ventricular mass. As conduction spreads slowly and abnormally through the ventricular mass, the QRS complex will becomes widened.

A wide QRS complex, also occurs if depolarization begins within the ventricle itself. For example, idioventricular rhythm or delay in the Purkinje system conduction.

Remember

Widening of the QRS indicates delayed and abnormal conduction through the ventricle due to any cause.

What is Bundle Branch Block (BBB)?

It is an electrocardiographic pattern that results either from delay or interruption of conduction through a bundle branch (right or left).

In normal heart, the time taken for the impulse to travel from interventricular septum to the ventricles is less than 0.12 sec (120 ms) which means three small squares (0.4 × 3) = 120 ms). If QRS duration is increased to more than 0.12 sec, then conduction through either one of the bundle or Purkinje fibers is delayed.

Remember

Normal QRS resulting from septal activation from left to right and then activation of the both the ventricles is less than 0.12 sec; the further lengthening of this QRS interval produces a bundle branch block pattern.

Right Bundle Branch Block (RBBB)

What is Right Bundle Branch Block?

The ECG pattern that results from interruption of conduction through the right bundle branch is called *right bundle branch block (RBBB)*. RBBB indicates problem in the right side of the heart. In some healthy people, incomplete RBBB pattern can be normal. Right bundle branch block can be congenital also.

It may be complete or incomplete. It is said to be *complete* if QRS duration is > 0.12 sec and *incomplete* when QRS duration is between 0.10 and 0.12 sec. The incomplete bundle branch block is now-a-days an absolute term.

Causes

1. *Congenital:* It is common in children.
2. *Acquired*
   - Coronary artery disease
   - Cardiomyopathies
   - Hypertensive heart disease
   - Congenital heart disease (ASD, VSD and Ebstein anomaly)
   - Acute massive pulmonary embolism
   - Myocarditis
   - Cardiac contusion
   - Phasic aberrant intraventricular conduction
   - Idiopathic

The electrocardiographic pattern (Figs 3.6 and 3.7)

1. The duration of QRS complex is $\geq$ 0.1 2 sec.
2. The shape of QRS in lead V_1 and V_2 is rSR′ (a morphology similar to 'rabbit ears') and qRS in leads I, aVL, V_5 and V_6. This occurs as follows:

    i. The initial r in V_1 and q in V_5 and V_6 is due to septal activation which proceed normally from left to right (Fig. 3.6, vector 1).

    ii. Now, due to block in the right bundle, the activation of left paraseptal region and free walls of left ventricle occurs. This is in contrast to normal, results in deep S

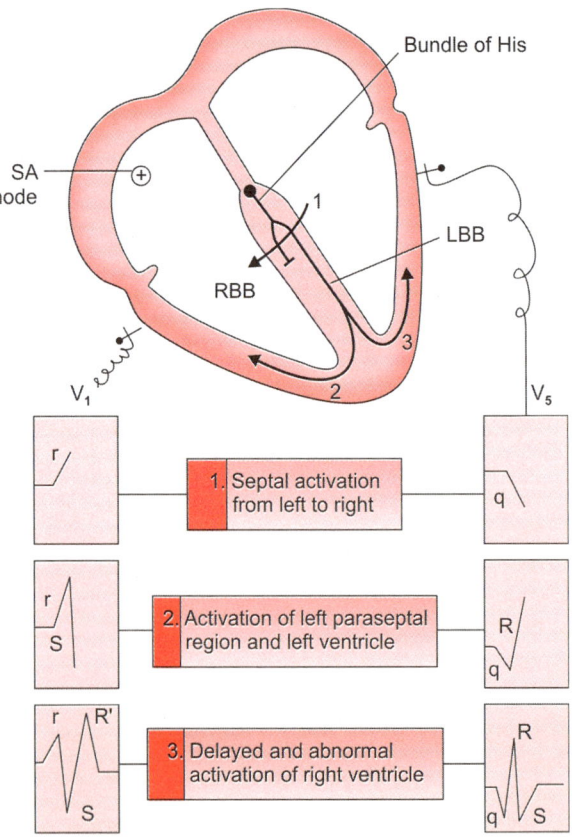

Fig. 3.6: Pathogenesis of right bundle branch block pattern

wave in V_1 and V_2 and a R wave in V_5–V_6 (Fig. 3.6, vector 2).

iii. Last of all, the right ventricle is activated by delayed and abnormal mechanism resulting in secondary R wave (R') in V_1 and a corresponding S in V_5–V_6 (Fig. 3.6, vector 3).

In this way rSR' pattern occurs in V_1 and qRS occurs in V_5–V_6 which is wider (> 0.12 sec) and abnormal.

3. The VAT is increased in leads V_1 and V_2.

Note: Normally, rSr' pattern can be seen where r' wave is small and rudimentary. This pattern occurs in 5% of normal persons.

4. The associated ST segment depression and T wave inversion occurs in leads V_1–V_2 secondary to abnormal intraventricular conduction. It is made clear that it is not due to myocardial involvement.

Remember

Wide rsR' or RSR' pattern > 0.12 sec in lead V_1 invariably indicates RBBB (Fig. 3.7).

Left Bundle Branch Block (LBBB)

What does LBBB Means?

Left bundle branch block is an ECG pattern that results either from delay or complete interruption of conduction through the left bundle branch resulting in delayed and abnormal activation of the left ventricle through right bundle. The QRS is > 0.12 sec.

Causes

It is rarely congenital, but always acquired. The common causes are:

1. Coronary artery disease.
2. Cardiomyopathy and myocarditis.
3. Hypertensive heart disease

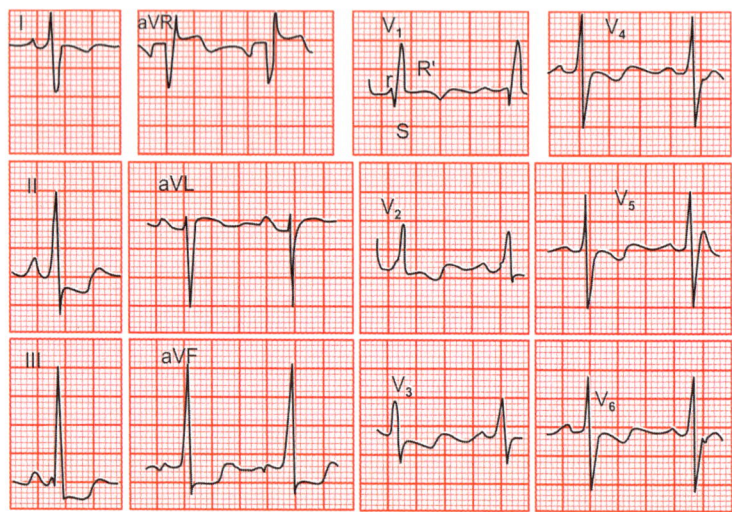

Fig. 3.7: Right bundle branch block (RBBB). The ECG shows (i) *Right axis deviation*; (ii) *Clockwise rotation* (deep S persists in V_5–V_6); (iii) *The rSR' pattern* (> 0.12 sec) in lead V_1 and deep wide S wave in V_5–V_6; (iv) *The ST depression and T wave inversion* in V_1 occurs due to RBBB. The generalised ST segment depression with inverted T is due to associated myocardial ischaemia

4. Aortic valve disease
5. Drugs, e.g. quinidine.

The electrocardiographic criteria (Figs 3.8 and 3.9)

The spread of excitation from SA node to AV node is normal, hence, P waves are normal.

1. *Absent Q waves in leads V_5–V_6, I and aVL:* Instead of normal left to right activation, the septum in LBBB is activated from right to left (R→L). This results in initial r wave instead of normal q wave in leads I, aVL, V_5 and V_6 with a corresponding q wave in leads V_1 or V_2; this being a very small is not seen (Fig. 3.8, vector 1).

☞ *Due to LBBB, there is no q wave in leads I, aVL and V_5–V_6.*

2. *Delayed and anomalous left septal and paraseptal activation:* The right paraseptal activation proceeds normally, occurs earlier than delayed and anomalous left paraseptal activation with

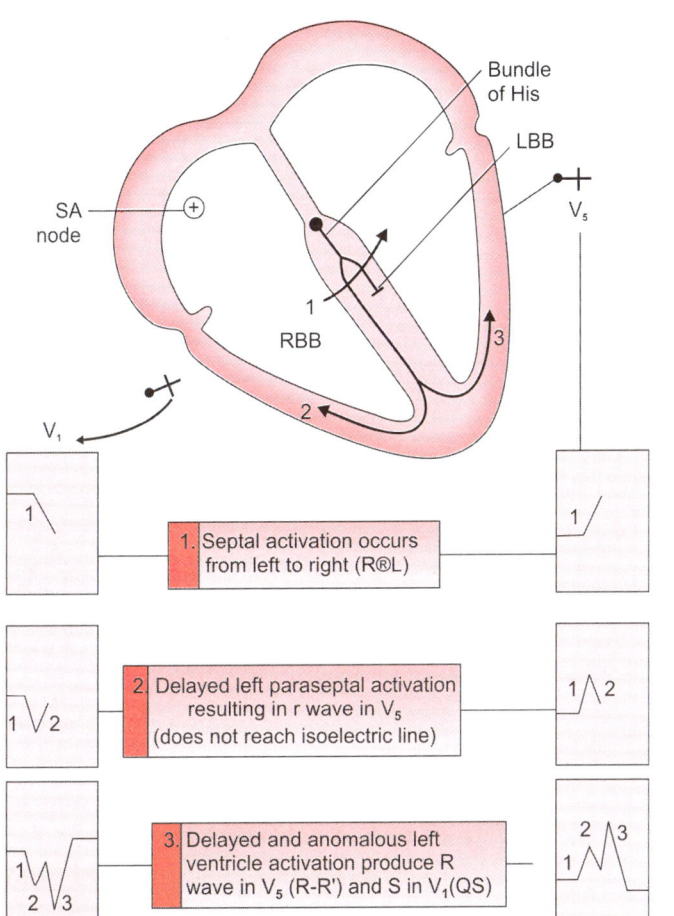

Fig. 3.8: Pathogenesis of left bundle branch block (LBBB) pattern

the result right ventricular activation precedes left ventricular activation resulting in small inscription of r wave in lead V_1 and a small S wave in lead V_5. These waves being too small do not reach isoelectric time, hence may produce a notch on the S wave in V_1 and on R wave in V_5 (Fig. 3.8, vector 2).

3. *Delayed and anomalous activation of left ventricle:* The left ventricle is activated in delayed and anomalous manner (Fig. 3.8, vector 3), resulting in a wide R wave in leads I, aVL, V_5

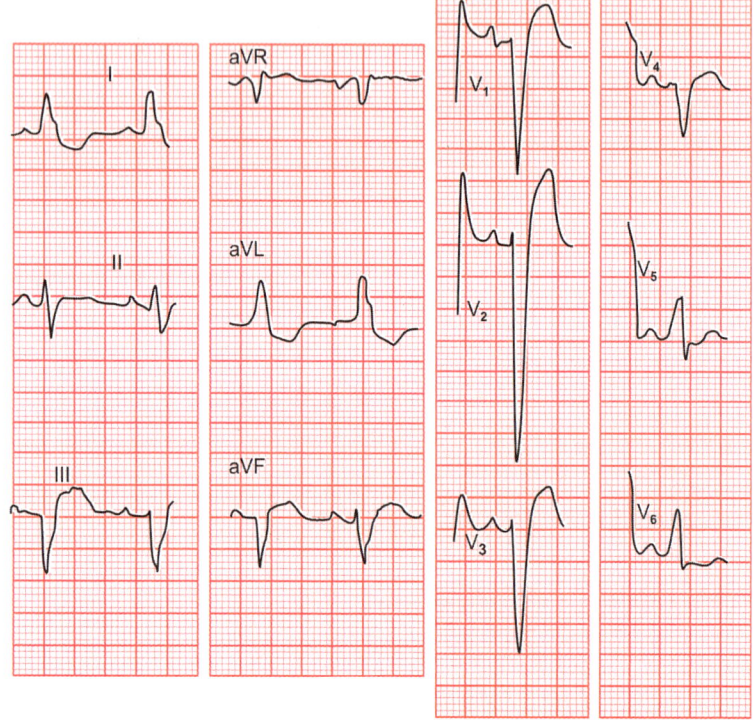

Fig. 3.9: Left bundle branch block. The ECG shows (i) *Left axis deviation*; (ii) *Loss of q waves* in leads I, aVL and V_5–V_6; (iii) *Wide slurred R* in V_5–V_6; (iv) *Wide QRS* > 0.12 sec in leads I, aVL, V_5 and V_6; (v) *Associated ST segment depression* in leads I, aVL, V_5–V_6 with T inversion

and V_6 and a corresponding deep S wave in right precordial leads (V_1–V_2).

In LBBB the morphology of QRS in leads V5–V6 is either a slurred R. RR′ or notched R or RSR′ pattern; and in lead V_1 there is QS pattern.

4. The VAT in left precordial leads is prolonged beyond 0.05 sec.

5. The associated ST segment depression and T wave inversion is seen in leads V_5–V_6.

These changes are secondary to conduction defect itself.

How to Diagnose the Bundle Branch Block?

The most useful leads to diagnose the bundle branch block are V_1 and V_6.

- Look at the leads V_1 and V_6. Is there is wide QRS > 0.12 sec? If yes:
- Now look at the pattern of QRS in lead V_1 and V_6 to decide whether bundle branch block is right or left (Read Table 3.1).

Table 3.1: Differentiating QRS pattern of BBB		
Leads	*RBBB*	*LBBB*
V_1	rSR'	QS
V_6	qRS	slurred R or RR' or RSR

FASCICULAR BLOCKS

The heart is considered to have three fascicles, i.e. the right bundle is considered as one fascicle and left bundle consists of other two fascicles called *left anterior fascicle* and *left posterior fascicle* (Fig. 3.10).

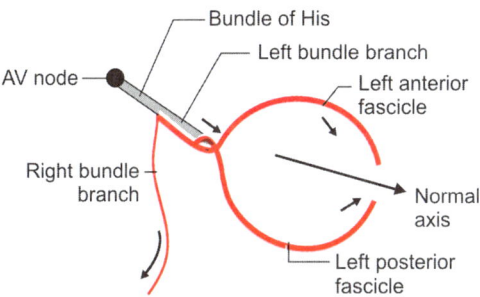

Fig. 3.10: The three fascicles (pathways) of the ventricular depolarisation. The spread of wave of excitation occurs along the arrows to depolarise both the ventricles simultaneously. The cardiac axis remains normal

Left Anterior Fascicular Block (LAFB)

Definition

A delay or block in conduction through anterior fascicle of left bundle is called *left anterior fascicular block* or *left anterior hemiblock*. The left anterior fascicle is long and thin and has single source of blood supply, hence, is more commonly involved than posterior fascicle.

Causes

1. Coronary artery disease.
2. Cardiomyopathies and myocarditis.
3. Long-standing systemic hypertension
4. Aortic valve disease
5. Congestive heart failure
6. Endocardial cushion defect (ostium premium defect).
7. Transient during infarction and arrhythmias.

The electrocardiographic criteria (Fig. 3.11)

Due to block or delay in left anterior fascicle, the excitation wave proceeds through the posterior fascicle, hence, postero-inferior portion (area supplied by the fascicle) of the left ventricle is activated first. Therefore, the initial QRS septal vector (vector 1, Fig. 3.11) is directed to the right (causing q wave in leads I and aVL) and inferiorly (causing R wave in leads II, III and aVF). Later the anterior fascicle is activated via Purkinje system resulting in a vector (vector 2, Fig. 3.11). Oriented to the left causing R wave in leads I and aVL (qR pattern is formed) and superiorly causing a S wave in leads II, III and aVF (rS pattern in these leads).

Due to differences in the orientation of the initial and terminal QRS vectors, the mean vector (vector 3, Fig. 3.11 remains to the left and superiorly producing left axis deviation of more than 30°. The duration of QRS remains normal.

ECG characteristics of LAFB (Fig. 3.12)

1. The duration of QRS is either normal or slightly prolonged but does not exceed 0.11 sec.
2. Left axis deviation > –30°.
3. A small q wave and tall R wave (qR pattern is seen in leads I and aVL.
4. A small r wave and deep S wave (rS pattern) is seen in leads II, III and aVF.

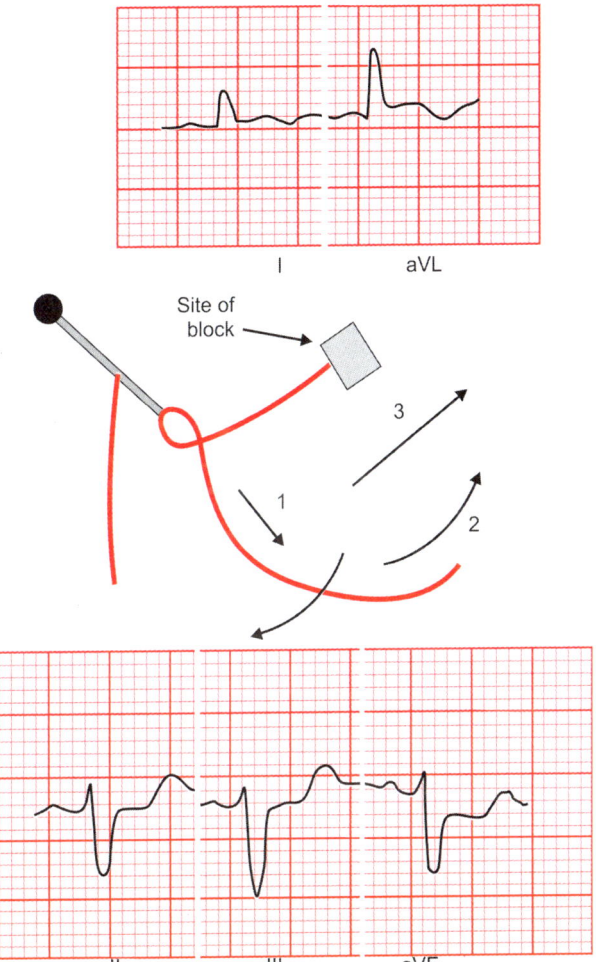

Fig. 3.11: Left anterior fascicular block. The mechanism of evolution of ECG pattern:

Vector 1: It is oriented to the right (produces q wave in lead I an aVL) and inferiorly (produces r wave in leads II, III and aVL)

Vector 2: Oriented to left and superiorly (produces S wave in leads II, III and aVF.

Vector 3: Resultant vector is oriented to the left producing left axis deviation > –30°

Remember

Left axis deviation > –30° is the hallmark of left anterior fascicular block.

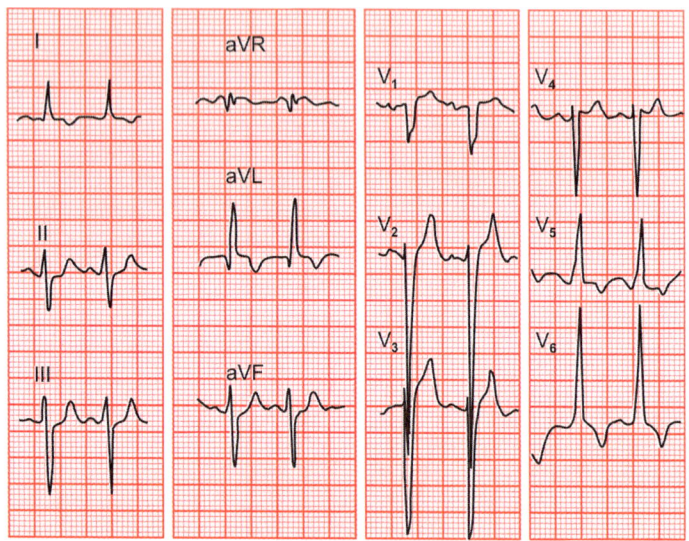

Fig. 3.12: Left anterior fascicular block. The ECG shows (i) QRS axis > –30°; (ii) There is rS pattern in leads II, III and aVF; (iii) The QRS duration is normal

Left Posterior Fascicular Block

Definition

A delay or block of conduction through the posterior fascicle of the left bundle is called "left posterior fascicular block".

Causes

1. Ischaemic heart disease.
2. Left ventricular hypertrophy.
3. Cardiomyopathy.
4. Cardiac surgery.

The electrocardiographs criteria (Fig. 3.13)

Due to block in the posterior fascicle, the excitation wave spreads through the anterior fascicle resulting in an initial vector (vector 1, Fig. 3.13) oriented to the left (causes R wave in lead I) and superiorly (causes Q waves in leads II, III and aVF). Later when the posterior fascicle is activated beyond

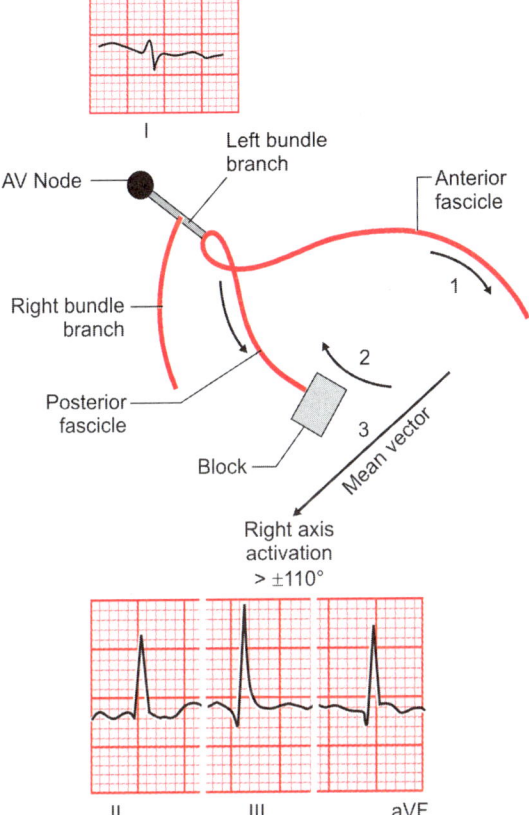

Fig. 3.13: Left posterior fascicular block (diagram). The mechanisms of evolution of ECG changes:

Vector 1: It is oriented to the left (R wave in lead I) and superiorly (Q waves in leads II, III and aVF).

Vector 2: It is oriented to the right (S wave in lead I) and inferiorly (R wave in leads II, III and aVF).

Vector 3: Mean vector is directed to right and inferiorly (right axis deviation > +110°.

the site of block via Purkinje system, the later vector (vector 2, Fig. 3.13) is oriented to the right (causes S wave in lead I) and inferiorly (causes R wave in leads II, III and aVF). The net result is right axis deviation from +110° to 180° usually $\geq$ +140°.

Remember

Right axis deviation > +110° is characteristic features of left posterior fascicular block provided other causes of right axis deviation have been ruled out such as RVH, RBBB, lateral wall infarction, cor pulmonale and acute pulmonary embolism.

The electrocardiographic characteristic of left posterior fascicular block (Fig. 3.14)

1. Right axis deviation > +110° (usually around + 140°)
2. There is rS pattern is lead I and qR pattern in leads II, III and aVF (Table 3.2).
3. The duration of QRS complex is slightly prolonged but does not exceed 0.11 sec.

Table 3.2: Summary of fascicular block		
	LAFB	*LPFB*
Axis	Left > −30°	Right > +110°
Lead I	qR pattern	rS pattern
Lead III	rS pattern	qR pattern

COMBINED BLOCKS

Bifascicular Block

- RBBB plus left anterior fascicular block.
- RBBB plus left posterior fascicular block.

The combination of RBBB with either left anterior fascicular or left posterior fascicular block is called *bifascicular block.*

Right bundle branch block with left anterior fascicular block (Fig. 3.15)

This is commonest type of bifascicular block. When the right bundle and left anterior fascicle are blocked, the ventricular activation takes place through midseptal and posterior fascicular fibres.

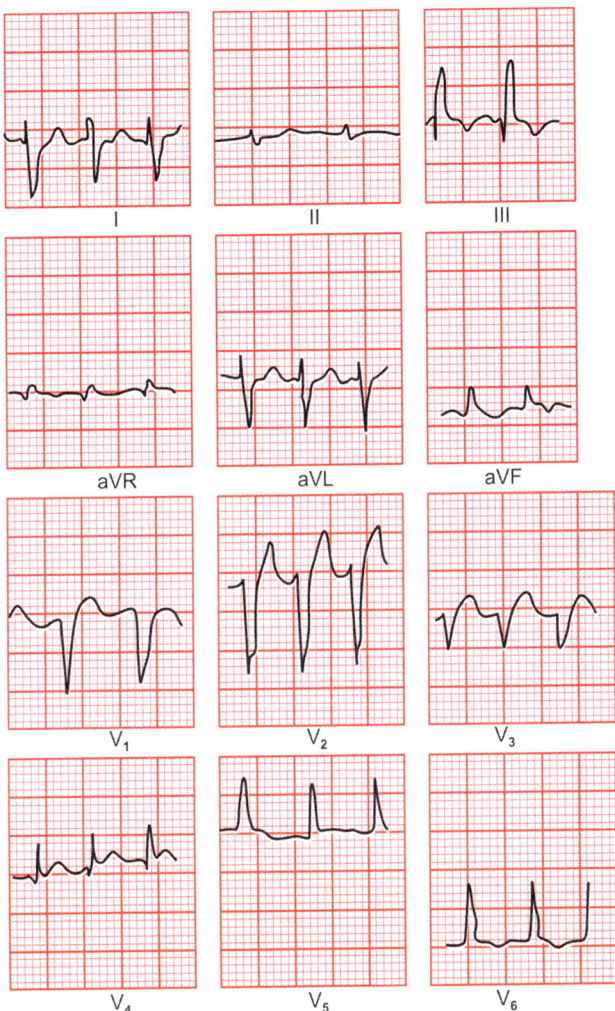

Fig. 3.14: Left posterior fascicular block. The electrocardiogram shows the following features (i) The means frontal QRS axis is + 140°; (ii) There is rS complex in leads I and aVL and qR complex in leads III and aVF; (iii) There is rS complex in leads V_1–V_3 with Rs in leads V_5–V_6; (iv) There is associated change in ST segment and T waves. The T waves are inverted in leads III and aVF and upright in leads I and aVL

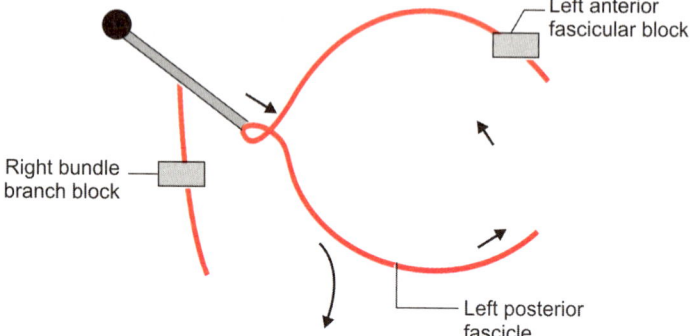

Fig. 3.15: Bifascicular block (diagram). In the presence of RBBB *plus* LAFB, the ventricular excitation wave spreads through posterior fascicle indicated by arrows

Causes

1. Atherosclerotic heart disease.
2. Hypertensive heart disease.
3. Cardiomyopathies.
4. A complication of heart surgery.
5. In association with myocardial infarction.
6. Idiopathic fibrosis of both mitral and aortic valve rings.
7. Congenital heart disease, e.g. septum primum ASD, endocardial cushion defect, single ventricle and Fallot tetralogy.

The ECG characteristics (Fig. 3.16)

1. *Right bundle branch block pattern:* A wide R wave or rSR′ pattern is seen in leads V_1 and V_2 with corresponding deep S wave —qRS pattern is seen in V_5–V_6.
2. *Left anterior fascicular block:* It will be projected as left axis deviation > −30° on frontal plane.

☞ *The pattern of RBBB plus left axis deviation invariably indicates a bifascicular block.*

Clinical significance

1. This type of bifascicular block carries a high-risk of going into complete heart block.

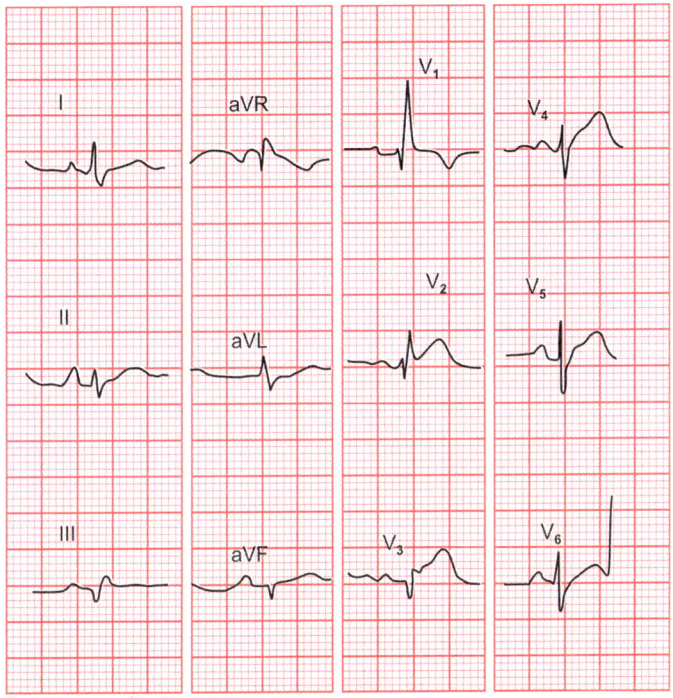

Fig. 3.16: Right bundle branch block with left anterior fascicular block (bifascicular block). The ECG shows (i) *Left anterior fascicular block*. There is left axis deviation of > –30° with rS pattern in leads II and III with deep S wave in lead III; (ii) The right bundle branch block. A wide rSR' pattern is seen in leads V_1–V_3 and *wide* S wave in V_4–V_6; (iii) *The ST-T changes of RBBB*, i.e. depression of ST segment and inversion of T wave is present in V_1

2. When this bifascicular block is present in a patient with myocardial infarction then the prognosis is bad because of two reasons:

    i. This type of bifascicular block indicates extensive myocardial damage.

    ii. There is high-risk of developing complete heart block.

Right bundle branch block with left posterior fascicular block

It is characterised by the presence of RBBB *plus* abnormal right axis deviation more than +110°. It is stressed here that right bundle branch block also shifts the axis to the right but not beyond +110°, hence, more than +110° right axis deviation constitutes posterior fascicular block in addition.

☞ *RBBB plus right axis deviation > +110° constitute a bifascicular block consisting of RBBB and left posterior fascicular block.*

ACCELERATED CONDUCTION OR PRE-EXCITATION

Definition

It is an electrocardiographic term used to denote rapid conduction through an anomalous (accessory) pathway resulting in pre-excitation (ventricular activation occurs earlier than expected).

Types

Two main types of accelerated conduction recognised on the ECG are:

1. *Wolff-Parkinson-White (WPW) conduction* (e.g. Kent bundle conduction). The rapid conduction is through Kent bundle (an accessory tract) which connects an atrium with a ventricle directly bypassing the AV node (Fig. 3.17).
2. *Lown-Ganong-Levine (LGL) conduction* (e.g. James bundle conduction). The rapid conduction occurs via James bundle (an accessory tract) that connects atrium with the bundle of His (atriohistian tract) bypassing the AV node (Fig. 3.17).

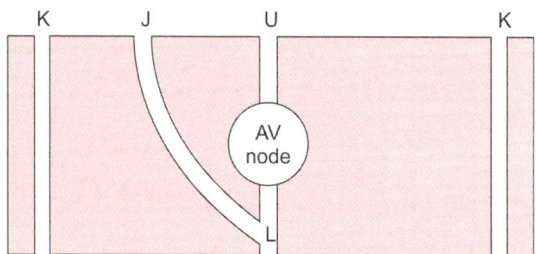

Fig. 3.17: Two common pathways of accelerated conduction K = Kent bundle that connects an atrium and the ventricle directly. J = James bundle connects atrium with the bundle of His. U = Upper common pathway, L = Lower common pathway

In accelerated conduction or pre-excitation, the AV node is bypassed by a tract called bypass tract or accessory pathway.

WOLFF-PARKINSON-WHITE (WPW) SYNDROME

Definition

It is an electrocardiographic syndrome that results from the conduction of the sinus or atrial impulses to the ventricles through normal and an anomalous pathways (Kent bundle) simultaneously.

The ECG characteristics (Figs 3.18A and B)

1. A short P-R interval < 0.12 sec.
2. QRS is widened and its duration is > 0.12 sec.
3. *Delta wave or pre-excitation wave:* This wave is seen as a notch or slur on the QRS deflection. It is seen on the ascending limb if the major deflection is upwards (Figs 3.18A and B) or on its descending limb if the major deflection is downwards.
4. Normal P-J interval.

Pathogenesis of WPW (Kent bundle conduction)

1. *Atrial activation:* It proceeds normal from SA node to atria resulting in normal P waves (Figs 3.19A and B).
2. *Ventricular premature excitation or pre-excitation:* In classic WPW syndrome (Kent bundle), the sinus beat or activation wave splits into two fronts; one follows the normal conduction pathways while the other passes rapidly through Kent bundle to reach the ventricle earlier than the front conducted through normal pathway. This is because accessory pathway does not delay the impulse; while AV node delays the other activation wave called *physiological delay*. The net result is short P-R interval.

☞ *A short P-R interval is due to rapid conduction through an accessory pathway.*

The activation wave conducted through the accessory pathway reaches one of the ventricles (ventricle connected with the pathway) earlier and excites it prematurely; the onward activation of the ventricles occur through the normal ordinary myocardial tissue which is poor and slow conducting medium than the highly specialised Purkinje

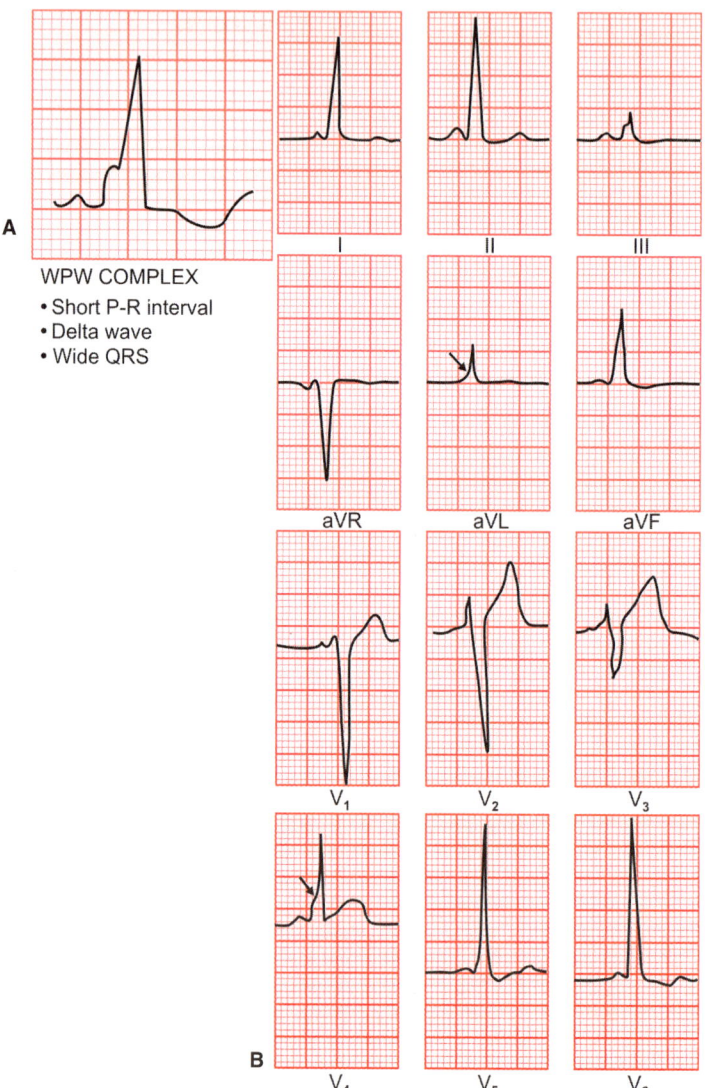

A

WPW COMPLEX
- Short P-R interval
- Delta wave
- Wide QRS

Figs 3.18A and B: Wolff-Parkinson-White (WPW) syndrome. (A) Diagrammatic illustration of basic electrocardiographic deflections. A P-QRS-T complex drawn shows a short P-R interval, a delta wave on the upstroke of R wave, wide QRS and normal. P-J interval; (B) The ECG shows a short P-R interval (< 10 sec), a positive delta wave on positive QRS (↑) in leads I, aVL and V₄–V₆. There is negative delta wave on negative QRS (↑) in leads aVR and V₁–V₃. The QRS is wide (> 0.12 sec). The ST-T vector is opposite to QRS, hence, the leads showing upright QRS have negative T waves and vice versa system. Pre-excitation is therefore slow and bizarre producing a delta wave, the amplitude of which varies with the size of myocardium depolarised (Fig. 3.19C).

3. *Terminal ventricular activation:* The ventricular activation initiated by preexcitation wave is completed by activation front that has passed normally through AV node. Thus, QRS deflection is wide and bizarre due to fusion of normal and abnormal activation fronts (Fig. 3.19D).

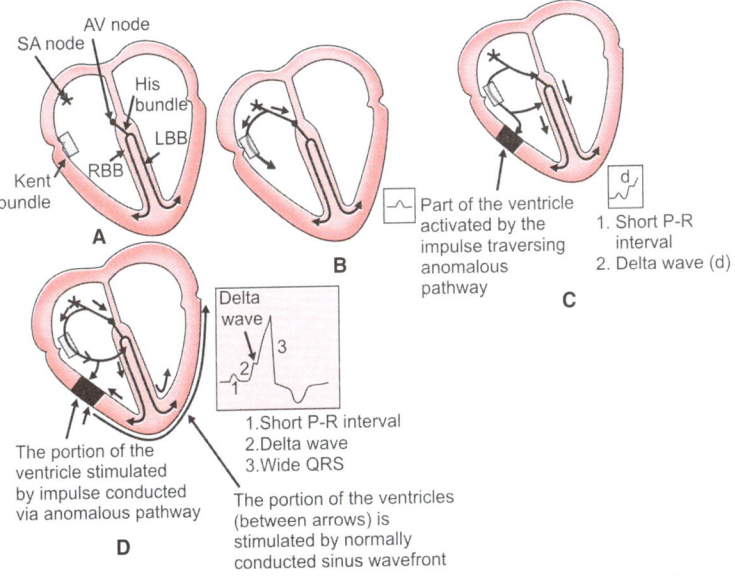

Figs 3.19A to D: WPW syndrome pathogenesis. (A) Normal anatomy of basic anomalous pathway; (B) Atrial activation producing a normal P wave; (C) Ventricular activation. A part of the ventricle is activated prematurely by a part of activation front that has traversed the anomalous tract to reach the ventricle earlier than normal sinus activation front. The short P-R interval and delta wave indicate premature excitation of ventricle through the accessory pathway; (D) Completed activation of ventricles). The unshaded part of the ventricles is activated by the normally conducted sinus impulse, thus ventricular activation process is completed leading to wide QRS

Intermittent WPW Conduction

The WPW may be regular but mostly is intermittent. In intermittent WPW syndrome, the complexes showing WPW type of conduction (short P-R interval, delta wave and wide bizarre QRS) are intermingled with normal conduction. It may occur periodically or may occur regularly.

Clinical significance

WPW type of conduction may result in:
1. Reciprocating tachycardia (wide QRS tachycardia).
2. Atrial fibrillation with fast conduction.

4

Disturbance of Cardiac Rhythm

- Intrinsic rhythmicity of the heart and natural pacemakers
- Normal sinus rhythm, sinus bradycardia and tachycardia
- Abnormal rhythms
  - Atrial
  - AV nodal/junctional
  - Ventricular

INTRINSIC RHYTHMICITY OF THE HEART

The SA node has an intrinsic property of the heart to generate a rhythm called normal pace or rhythm of the heart at a rate of 72–80 beats / min. When rhythm begins in the SA node. the heart is said to be in sinus rhythm. When the rhythm starts from a place other than SA node, it is called an *arrhythmia*.

What are Natural Pacemaker of the Heart and their Rates?

The pacemaker cells are present throughout the conduction system (SA node, atria, AV node, bundle of His and ventricles) but their discharge rate varies due to their inherent property More distally a pacemaker is situated from SA node, the slower is its inherent rate of discharge. This is the reason that ventricular pacemaker produces lowest heart rate. The discharge rates of various pacemaker may be written in descending orders as follows:

SA node > AV node > bundle of His > ventricle.

The potential pacemakers are represented in Fig. 4.1 and their discharge rates are given in Box 1.

NORMAL AND ABNORMAL RHYTHM

The rate and rhythm of the heart is controlled by SA node which is dominant pacemaker. The SA node is the fastest pacemaker

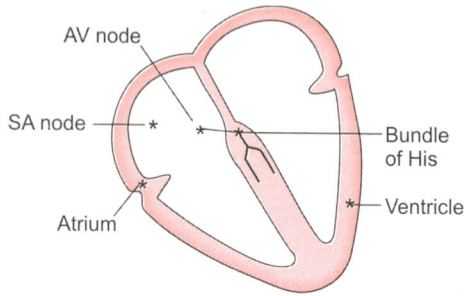

Fig. 4.1: Pacemaker sites in the heart

BOX 1: DISCHARGE RATE OF PACEMAKER	
Pacemaker	*Discharge rate per minute*
1. SA node	60–80 approx
2. AV node	50–60 approx
3. Bundle of His	40–50 approx
4. Purkinje fibers (ventricle)	15–40 approx

and suppresses the other pacemakers (subsidiary pacemakers), giving the wrong impression that there is only one pacemaker of the heart. It is an inherent property of the heart that when a pacemaker fails, then a subsidiary pacemaker situated next to it takes over the control of cardiac rhythm. For example, if SA node fails or defaults, the AV node takes over the control with discharge rate of 50–60/min. The rhythm produced by AV node pacemaker is called *nodal rhythm*, which is called an escape rhythm because AV node has escaped from the control of SA node. Therefore, presence of AV nodal rhythm indicates failure of SA node.

AV nodal escape rhythm is abnormal rhythm and indicates failure of normal sinus rhythm.

In case AV node fails to conduct the sinus beats (complete heart block), the control of the cardiac rhythm is taken by either bundle of His or ventricular myocardium producing abnormal idionodal or idioventricular rhythm respectively.

Types of abnormal rhythms (Fig. 4.2)

Depending on the site of origin, the abnormal rhythm is divided in two types:

1. *Supraventricular rhythm:* It originates from any site above the bundle of His. It includes abnormal rhythms from atria and AV node (Figs 4.2A). In supraventricular rhythms, the depolarisation (excitation) wave spreads to the ventricle via normal pathway, i.e. through His bundle, bundle branches and the ventricles. The QRS complex is therefore normal and is the same whether depolarisation is initiated by the SA node, or atria or the AV node (Fig. 4.28).

> *An abnormal rhythm with narrow QRS complex is invariously supraventricular rhythm.*

2. *Ventricular rhythm:* In the ventricular rhythm, the depolarisation wave (wave of excitation) spreads through the ventricular myocardium or Purkinje fibers which is slow and poor conducting tissue, hence, the QRS complex is wide and bizarre (Fig. 4.2C). Repolarisation is also abnormal, so the T wave is of abnormal shape (inverted).

> *Wide QRS rhythm refers to an abnormal rhythm originating from the bundle branches or ventricular myocardium or there is retrograde conduction through the ventricle.*

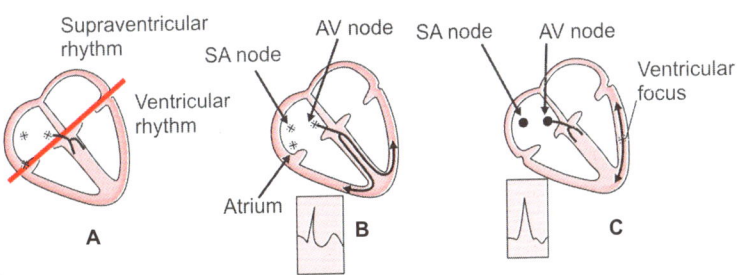

Figs 4.2A to C: Abnormal rhythms. (A) Division of abnormal rhythms into two main types; supraventricular and ventricular; (B) Spread of excitation (depolarisation) in supraventricular rhythm (e.g. origin in SA node, atria and AV node is represented by a star). The QRS is narrow and normal; (C) Spread of excitation in ventricular rhythm (focus indicated by a star). The QRS is wide

What is Sinus Rhythm?

Rhythm is said to be sinus when impulses originating from the SA node are conducted to the ventricles via AV node. It is a normal rhythm.

The ECG characteristics

1. *The P wave is normal:* It is upright in all standard leads except aVR. It is also upright in precordial leads except V_1 where it may he biphasic.
2. The P-P and R-R intervals remain constant.
3. The heart rate ranges between 60 and 100 bpm.
4. There is no ectopic activity.

What is Sinus Arrhythmia?

Changes in the heart rate associated with respiration are normally seen in young people, and this is called *"sinus arrhythmias"*. Heart rate increases during inspiration and slows during expiration. In diseased state, the sinus arrhythmia can be non-respiratory (Fig. 4.3).

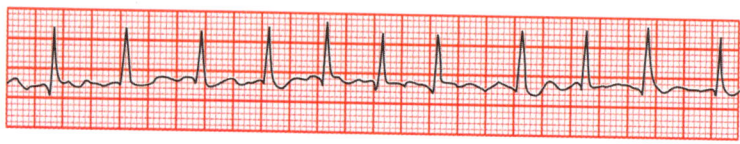

Fig. 4.3: Non-respiratory sinus arrhythmia

What is Sinus Bradycardia?

It is defined as sinus rhythm with a rate less than 60/min in an adult.

Causes

1. Physiological, i.e. vagotonic person, athletes and during sleep.
2. Hypothyroidism (myxoedema).
3. Obstructive jaundice.
4. Hypothermia.
5. Sick sinus syndrome.
6. Electrolyte disturbance, i.e. hyperkalaemia, hypermagnesaemia, etc.
7. Inferior wall infarction.
8. Drugs (digoxin, beta blockers and calcium channel blockers).
9. Second degree AV block (Mobitz II).
10. Raised intracranial tension.
11. Uraemia.

12. Poisoning (OP compounds, scorpion sting bite, etc.).
13. Hyperactive carotid sinus.

The electrocardiographic characteristics (Fig. 4.4)

1. Sinus rate < 60/min.
2. The P wave is normal and precedes each normal QRS complex.
3. The R-R interval is constant, but sinus arrhythmia often coexist with bradycardia.

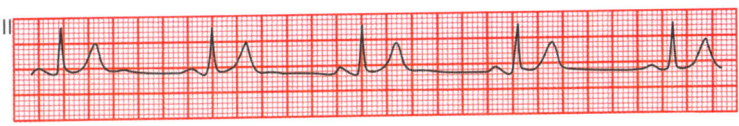

Fig. 4.4: Sinus bradycardia. The R-R interval is 30 mm, thus HR = 1500 ÷ 30 = 50/min

What do you Mean by Sinus Tachycardia?

It is defined as sinus rhythm with a heart rate equal to or greater than 100 beats/minute in an adult. During sinus tachycardia, the sinus node can exhibit a discharge rate between 100–180/min with extreme exertion.

Causes

1. Anxiety states, excessive use of tea, coffee, smoking, etc.
2. Hyperthyroidism.
3. Acute pulmonary embolism.
4. Congenital heart disease.
5. Drug induced (adrenaline, thyroid hormone prep, nicotine or alcohol, atropine, caffeine, amylnitrate, nifedipine, etc.).
6. Physiological in neonates and during REM sleep.

The ECG characteristics (Fig. 4.5)

1. Heart rate is generally > 100/min. The P-P intervals are constant but may vary slightly.
2. The P wave has normal configuration and precedes each narrow QRS with a stable P-R interval.
3. The R-R interval is also regular.
4. The QRS complexes are narrow.

V₃ (Two strips)

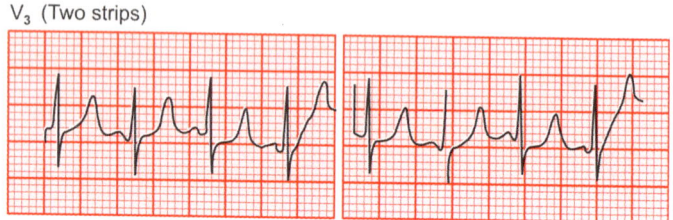

Fig. 4.5: Sinus tachycardia. The R-R interval is 11 mm, thus HR = 1500 ÷ 11 = 136/min

How to Describe an Abnormal Rhythm?

Three things are to be described

1. *Site of origin,* e.g. SA node, atria, AV node or ventricle. They are recognised by their characteristics.
2. *Discharge sequence:* Every rhythm has a discharge sequence such as normal sinus rhythm or an escape rhythm or idio-ventricular rhythm. Bradycardia, tachycardia, extrasystole, flutter and fibrillation also indicate the discharge sequence of a rhythm.
3. *Conduction ratio:* It is a ratio of total P waves to conducted P wave such as 2 : 1.3 : 1, etc. The first number indicate the number of P waves or F waves and the later indicates the number of conducted P or F.

How Would you Detect an Abnormal Rhythm?

Analysis of Cardiac Rhythm

The points to be analysed for normal or abnormal cardiac rhythm include:

1. Define the P wave and analyse it to know whether it is a normal P wave or abnormal P wave (ectopic, flutter or fibrillatory wave).
2. Calculate the atrial rate and ventricular rate. Normally, they are constant and equal.
3. Determine whether the P-P intervals and R-R intervals are regular or irregular. Normally, they are regular.
4. The relationship of P wave to QRS complex. Whether it is associated (P wave and QRS have constant relation); or dissociated (P has no relation to QRS) rhythm. Normally,

there is one P wave that precedes each QRS with fixed P-R interval.

5. Note the shape and width of QRS complex, i.e. narrow or wide. Normally, QRS is narrow.
6. Presence of ectopic activity: Normally, there is no premature or escape complex.

How do the Arrhythmias Originate (Arrhythmogenesis)?

The origin of abnormal cardiac rhythm is divided into two main groups.

I. *Abnormal automaticity:* The arrhythmia produced by accelerated automaticity are:
   - Sinus tachycardia
   - Escape rhythms
   - Accelerated AV nodal rhythm.
   - Ventricular tachyarrhythmias triggered by prolonged QT
   - Digitalis induced arrhythmias.

II. *Re-entry (circus movement)* (Figs 4.6A and B)
   Tachyarrhythmias due to re-entry mechanism are:
      i. Sinus node re-entrant tachycardia
     ii. Atrial flutter or fibrillation
    iii. Paroxysmal supraventricular tachycardia:
       - AV nodal re-entrant tachycardia (AVNRT)
       - Atrioventricular tachycardia (AVRT)
       - Pre-excitation syndrome with tachycardia (reciprocal tachycardia).

   IV. Ventricular tachycardia and ventricular fibrillation (Fig. 4.6B).

ATRIAL ARRHYTHMIAS

Atrial Ectopics (Premature beats or extrasystoles)

Atrial premature complex (APC) or a beat (APB) or an ectopic or an extrasystole is a premature discharge from an ectopic focus located somewhere in the atria outside the SA node.

Causes

- Sometimes a normal finding.
- Anxiety, stress, tea, coffee and alcohol intake.

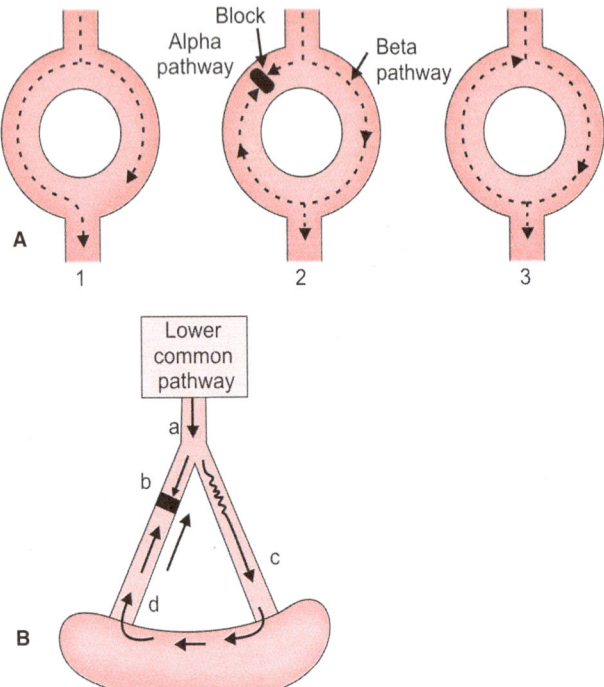

Figs 4.6A and B: Mechanisms of re-entry (circus movement). (A) Re-entrant supraventricular arrhythmia. (1) Shows the impulses passing down both limbs of the potential tachycardia circuit. (2) Shows that impulse is blocked in alpha pathway but proceeds slowly down the beta pathway and returns along the alpha pathway. (3) Shows the impulse travels so slowly along the beta pathway that when it returns along the alpha pathway to its starting point, it is able to travel down the beta pathway producing a circus movement tachycardia; (B) Re-entrant ventricular tachycardia (anatomical re-entry). The Purkinje fibers splits into two pathways. An impulse travelling through lower common pathway (a), gets blocked in antegrade conduction at site (b) (arrow followed by bar), but travels down slowly at (c) (serpentine arrow) to excite the ventricle. The impulse now re-enters the Purkinje system of myocardium, excites it and then re-enters at site (d) as a result of which ventricular extrasystole results. Continued re-entry in this manner produces ventricular tachycardia

- Heart disease such as heart failure, myocardial ischemia, valvular heart disease and coronary artery disease.
- Hyperthyroidism.
- COPD and chronic cor pulmonale.

- Systemic infections.
- Electrolyte disturbance, e.g. hypokalaemia.
- Digitalis toxicity.

The ECG characteristics (Figs 4.7A and B)

1. *The R-R intervals is intermittently irregular* due to interposition of an ectopic.
2. The *shape of P wave* of an atrial ectopic is different than normal sinus P.
3. *Fixed coupling interval (pre-ectopic interval):* The interval between a sinus beat and the APC is short and fixed also called pre-ectopic interval.
4. *A compensatory pause or postectopic interval* follows an atrial premature complex (APC) or an ectopic beat.
5. The *premature P wave may precede or follow or may get merged within QRS* (P is invisible) depending on the conduction into the ventricles.
6. The *shape of QRS* of an atrial premature complex is narrow.

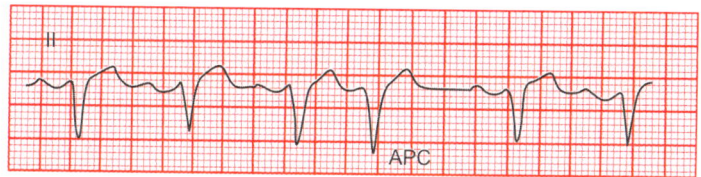

Fig. 4.7A: Atrial premature complexes (APCs). One APC is seen in lead II. The P wave of APC is not visible (i.e. embedded in QRS). APC is recognised by its early arrival than expected, i.e. short pre-ectopic interval

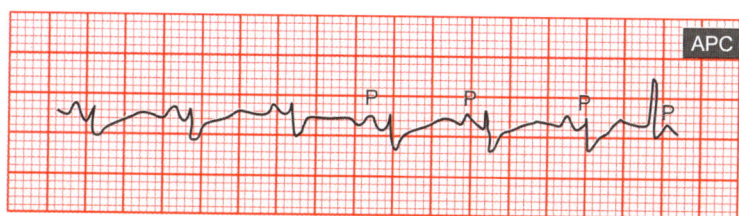

Fig. 4.7B: Atrial premature complexes (APCs). First 6 complexes are normal, i.e. P wave is followed by QRS. Last complex is an APC in which P wave follows QRS as it reaches later

7. The P-R interval of an APC may be short, normal, prolonged or absent. The length of P-R depends on the ability of the AV node to conduct an atrial ectopic to ventricles.

The best leads for assessment of atrial arrhythmia are leads II, III and aVF.

Atrial Escape Beat

Sometimes, an atrial premature complex (APC) may penetrate the SA node and reset its timing, and in the meantime, occasionally, an another APC instead of normal sinus beat may follow and this APC after a long interval is called an *atrial escape beat*. The atrial premature beat is inscribed late and does not have a compensatory pause; while an APC occurs early and is followed by a compensatory pause (read compensatory pause in ventricular arrhythmias).

☞ How to recognise an APC?

1. *Look at the rhythm strip and find out the premature complex by its early arrival than expected (short pre-ectopic interval).*

2. *Now analyse the complex: If an abnormal P or no P wave precedes a narrow QRS, the complex is an atrial premature complex (APC).*

Atrial Tachycardia

Atrial tachycardia is a supraventricular or narrow QRS tachycardia originating in the atria outside the SA node at a rate between 150 and 250 beats/min. Atrial tachycardia (non-paroxysmal) is frequently digitalis induced.

Causes

1. Digitalis toxicity
2. Valvular (rheumatic) heart disease
3. Coronary artery disease
4. Electrolyte imbalance
5. Cor pulmonale
6. Idiopathic.

The ECG characteristics (Figs 4.8A and B)

1. The P-P and R-R intervals are constant. Atrial and ventricular rates are between 150 and 250/min.
2. Each P wave is followed by a narrow QRS (1:1 conduction). However, conduction ratio can be 2:1 or more (two or more P waves for one QRS complex with an isoelectric baseline between P waves) especially in the presence of digitalis toxicity. This is called atrial tachycardia (nonparoxysmal) with AV block.
3. The P-R interval is short where P wave is seen nicely and conduction ratio is 1:1.
4. The shape of the P wave is often different from the normal sinus P wave. At faster rates, the abnormal P wave may be difficult to see or localise but it may distort the T wave of preceding beat, therefore, examine the preceding T wave carefully for any distortion.
5. The shape of the QRS is narrow, hence, also called *narrow QRS tachycardia*.
6. Atrial tachycardia may occur in paroxysm; when it terminates, a long pause is produced before normal sinus rhythm is resumed.
7. ST-T changes (the ST segment depression and T wave inversion) may appear in those leads having dominant upright QRS complexes. These indicate relative ischaemia due to tachycardia itself (*tachycardia induced ST-T changes*).

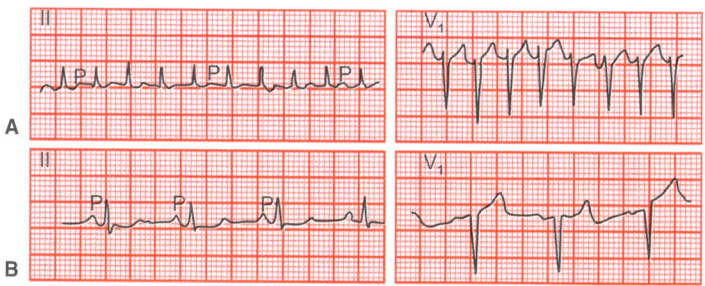

Figs 4.8A and B: Paroxysmal atrial tachycardia. (A) *Before reversion* (upper strip leads II and V$_1$). Heart rate is 183/min and regular. The QRS complexes are narrow. The P waves are nicely seen preceding the QRS especially in the lead II; (B) *After reversion*, the heart rate is 94/min and regular. The P waves are now clearly visible

Atrial Flutter

Atrial flutter is a supraventricular arrhythmia characterised by rapid and regular atrial rate between 250 and 350 bpm. The flutter (F) waves instead of normal P waves produce a *saw-tooth appearance* of baseline. It is commonly due to atrial re-entry (circus movement within atria).

Causes

1. Thyrotoxicosis
2. Valvular heart disease (rheumatic)
3. Ischaemic heart disease
4. Pericarditis (chronic)
5. Acute pulmonary embolism
6. Severe pulmonary disease
7. Congenital heart disease
8. Pre-excitation syndrome
9. Idiopathic.

The ECG characteristics (Figs 4.9 and 4.10)

1. *The normal P waves are absent:* Instead of P waves, there are flutter (F) waves. They assume *saw-tooth appearance*, nicely seen in inferior leads (II, III and aVF).
2. *The F waves are contiguous* due to continued atrial activity and there is no visible isoelectric line between them. Some F waves may be obscured by the QRS complex. Sometimes F waves may be equal to small QRS (Fig. 4.9).

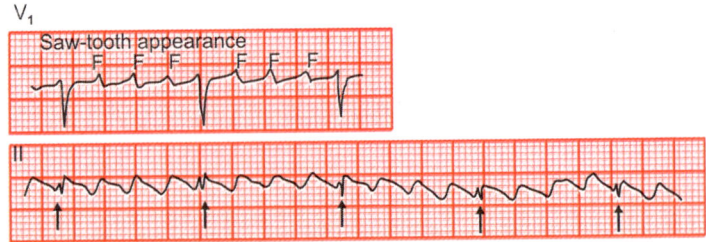

Fig. 4.9: Atrial flutter. Lead V_1 shows saw-tooth appearance. The heart rate is 62/min and atrial rate as 248/min indicating 4:1 conduction. The flutter waves in lead II are equal to QRS (↑) in the lower strip

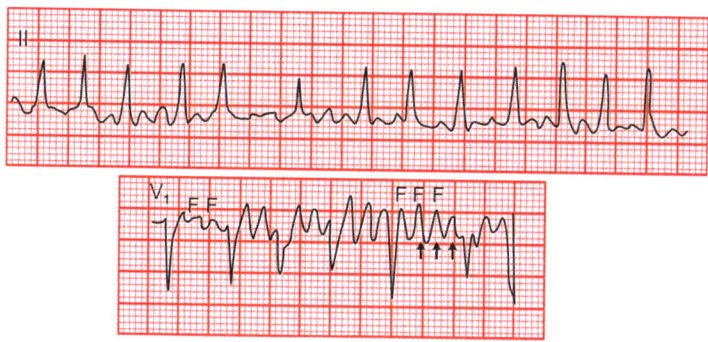

Fig. 4.10: Atrial flutter fibrillation. Note the large flutter (F) waves in leads II and V₁. The R-R interval is variable from beat-to-beat, hence it is flutter fibrillation instead of pure atrial flutter. The F waves in V₁ are as big as giant P waves and are more or less equal to QRS indicated by (↑)

3. The atrial rate varies between 250 and 350/min.
4. The ventricular rate is slow than atrial rate. This is because, AV node cannot conduct so many impulses. Normally, the AV node is unable to conduct more than 200 beats/min with the result, a physiological block develops to prevent transmission of these impulses.
5. The R-R interval is mostly regular due to fixed block but varies if block is variable.
6. The conduction ratio (ratio of F waves to a QRS complex) is usually an even and multiple of two (2:1, 4:1, 6:1) but can be odd (3:1). One-to-one conduction ratio (1:1) is rare.
7. The QRS complex is narrow and normal.

> ☞ *Saw-toothed, regular, identically recurring flutter waves called 'F' waves seen at a rate of about 300/min suggest atrial flutter.*

Atrial Fibrillation (AF)

It is a supraventricular arrhythmia characterised by replacement of P waves by fibrillatory (f) waves occurring at a rate varying between 350 and 600/min. The ventricular rate is irregular.

Causes

The causes are given in Box 2

BOX 2: CAUSES OF ATRIAL FIBRILLATION	
Common	**Uncommon**
• Rheumatic heart disease, e.g. mitral stenosis and mitral regurgitation	• Constrictive pericarditis
	• Cor pulmonale
	• Congenital heart disease, e.g. ASD and Ebstein's anomaly
• Thyrotoxicosis (thyrotoxic heart disease)	• WPW syndrome
• Coronary artery disease	• Left atrial myxoma
• Hypertensive heart disease	• Heart surgery
• Cardiomyopathies and diphtheric myocarditis	• Idiopathic (lone atrial fibrillation)

The ECG characteristics (Figs 4.11A and B)

1. *Fibrillatory (f) waves replace the normal P waves:* Instead of normal P waves, fibrillatory (f) waves are present, which causes undulation of the baseline (the baseline is wavy).

2. *Varying R-R interval:* Heart rate (ventricular rate) is irregularly irregular and the R-R interval is variable from beat-to-beat due to variable conduction through AV node.

3. *Morphology of QRS:* The QRS complexes are narrow due to normal intraventricular conduction.

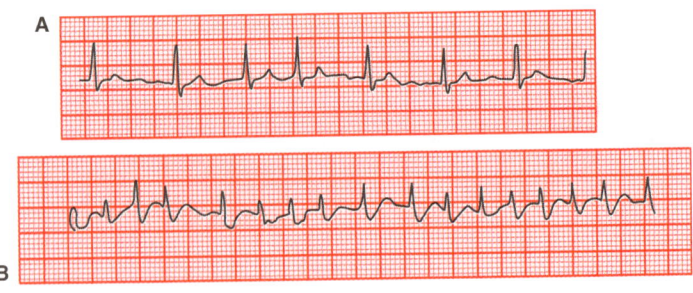

Figs 4.11A and B: Atrial fibrillation. (A) Fine atrial fibrillation. There is fine undulation of baseline with variable R-R intervals. The shape of QRS also changes. The heart rate is also slow, i.e. 90/min; (B) Fast atrial fibrillation. There is variable R-R intervals with undulating baseline and fast ventricular response (HR > 180/min approx). The fibrillatory waves are not visible

4. *Atrial rate is very high* varying between (350 and 600 beats/min.) but the ventricular rate is either one-fourth or half of it due to physiological block at AV node.

> ☞ *The presence of fibrillatory (F) waves, undulations of the baseline, irregular R-R intervals and rapid ventricular rate are diagnostic clues to atrial fibrillation.*

ATRIOVENTRICULAR (AV) NODAL DISTURBANCE

As already discussed, the SA node is dominant pacemaker—*"the king of his own Empire"*, suppresses all other subsidiary pacemakers, therefore, the AV nodal beats/rhythm occur secondary to involvement of SA node either by disease or by default. The nodal ectopics may also occur occasionally when the rate of SA node falls below the intrinsic discharge rate of AV node (e.g. in bradycardia or sinus arrhythmia).

The ECG characteristics of nodal beat/rhythm

1. The nodal impulse or impulses are conducted antegradely to the ventricles through the normal pathways and retrogradely to the atria producing *inverted P (P') waves in leads II, III and aVF with upright P wave in aVR*. The inverted P waves usually precede the QRS or may get burried within QRS, or rarely may follow QRS (Figs 4.12A to C).
2. *The QRS complexes are normal* due to normal intraventricular conduction.

AV Nodal Ectopics (Junctional ectopics)

The AV nodal ectopics are premature discharges from AV node occurring occasionally or intermittently. These are actually AV nodal escape beats because they occur when SA node has defaulted or may occur by usurpation.

Causes

1. Acute myocardial infarction (e.g. inferior wall infarction).
2. Heart failure.
3. Valvular heart disease (mitral or tricuspid).
4. Sick sinus syndrome.
5. Myocarditis and cardiomyopathies.

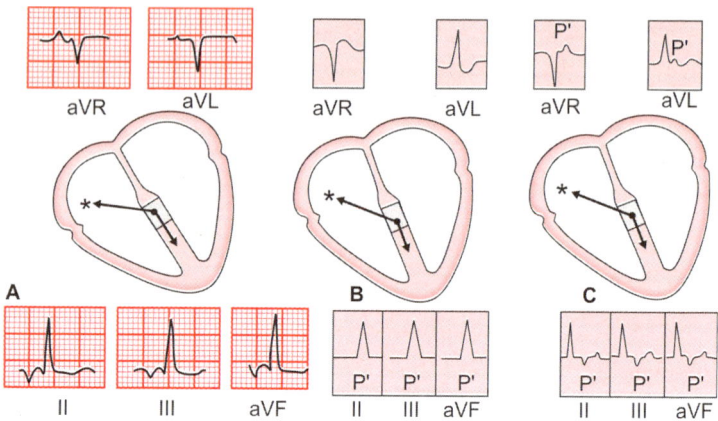

Figs 4.12A to C: Various conduction mechanisms and relation of P' waves to QRS in AV nodal beats/rhythm (leads II, III, aVR, aVL and aVF drawn). (A) It illustrates AV nodal beats with earlier retrograde conduction to the atria than antegrade conduction to the ventricles resulting in inverted P' waves (II,. III and aVF) preceding normal QRS; (B) It illustrates simultaneous and synchronous retrograde atrial and antegrade ventricular activation resulting in P' waves burried within QRS; (C) It illustrates the antegrade ventricular activation (conduction) earlier than retrograde atrial activation resulting in inverted P waves following the QRS in leads II, III and aVF

Note: If P wave is inverted in leads II, III and aVF then P will be upright in leads aVR and aVL. This is due to superior orientation of P wave vector

6. Drug effect (digitalis and theophylline).
7. Electrolyte disturbance.

The ECG characteristics (Figs 4.13 and 4.14)

1. *P wave morphology:* The P wave is inverted in leads II, III and aVF but upright in aVR. The inverted P may proceed, may get merged or may follow QRS.
2. *The P-R interval of an ectopic varies* (short or absent).
3. The *QRS is normal.*
4. *Fixed coupling interval* also called *pre-ectopic interval.* (An interval between the sinus beat and AV nodal ectopic.)
5. *Compensatory pause* also called post-ectopic interval. A postectopic compensatory pause follows an AV nodal ectopics but is absent in AV nodal escape beat/beats. (These beats come later than expected time.) The compensatory pause is longer than pre-ectopic interval, i.e. it confirms premature arrival of an ectopic.

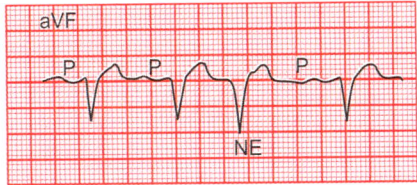

Fig. 4.13: Nodal ectopics (NE). One ectopic (labelled NE) is seen which has P wave embedded within QRS (P wave is not visible). There is a short coupling interval and a long compensatory pause following the ectopic

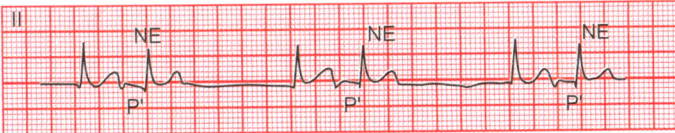

Fig. 4.14: Nodal bigeminy. The each sinus beat is followed by a nodal ectopic (NE) having an inverted P' and narrow QRS in a regular fashion

Remember

A nodal beat cannot have an upright P wave in leads II, III and aVF

AV Nodal Rhythm

AV nodal rhythm is usually an escape rhythm, occurs either by default or usurpation. The rate of this rhythm is the actual inherent rate of AV nodal discharge, i.e. 40–60/min.

Causes

1. High vagal tone—a normal phenomenon.
2. It is an escape rhythm occurring following profound bradycardia (slow SA node discharge).
3. It can appear during heart blocks.
4. Sick sinus syndrome.

The ECG characteristics (Fig. 4.15)

1. *Ventricular rate is regular* at a rate of 40–60 beats/min. The R-R intervals are regular.
2. Usually, the *P waves are not seen* because they are merged within QRS. At times, the *inverted P waves* may precede or follow QRS complexes.

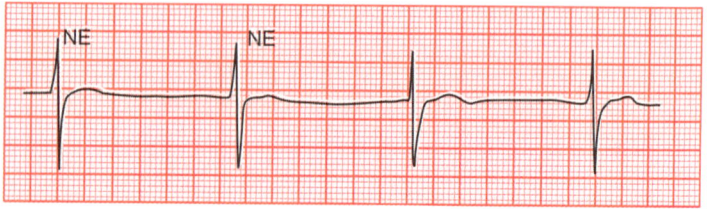

Fig. 4.15: Nodal rhythm at a rate of 43/min approx. There is no visible P waves which are embedded within QRS which is slightly wider than normal

3. *The QRS complexes are narrow* due to normal intraventricular conduction.

> ☞ *A regular rhythm at a rate of 40–60 bpm with no visible P wave is suggestive of AV nodal rhythm.*

Accelerated AV Nodal Rhythm or Idionodal Tachycardia

The AV node can accelerate its rate beyond its inherent rate of 40–60 bpm and may take the full control of the heart. This is an escape rhythm.

I. When the heart rate (ventricular rate) lies between 60 and 100 bpm (usual is 70–80 bpm), it is called *accelerated AV nodal rhythm* (Fig. 4.16).

II. When the heart rate becomes more than 100 bpm, then it is called *idionodal tachycardia*.

Causes

1. Digitalis toxicity
2. Acute rheumatic fever
3. Valvular heart disease

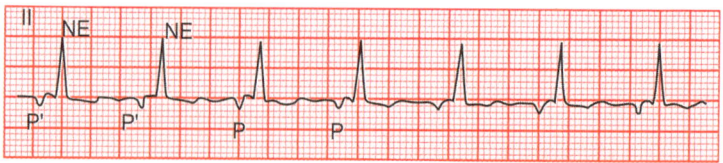

Fig. 4.16: Accelerated nodal rhythm. The lead II (rhythm strip) shows each complex has an inverted P(P') wave followed by a narrow QRS and upright T wave indicating a nodal beat. There are 7 such beats in a row constituting a nodal rhythm. The heart rate is about 83/min indicating accelerated nodal rhythm

4. Myocardial infarction
5. Heart failure
6. Myocarditis

The ECG characteristics

1. *Heart rate:* It lies between 70 and 80 bpm in accelerated nodal rhythm and may go beyond 100 bpm in idionodal tachycardia.
2. *The QRS complexes are narrow* but slightly wider than sinus complexes.
3. *AV dislocation:* It commonly occurs because its rate is just in the range of normal sinus rate. It may result in frequent capture and fusion complexes.

PAROXYSMAL SUPRAVENTRICULAR TACHYCARDIA

Paroxysmal supraventricular tachycardia (PSVT) is defined as conduction of supraventricular impulses at a rate > 100 bpm with narrow QRS, regular R-R intervals and without an evidence of pre-excitation. If it is associated with wide QRS, then it is called PSVT with aberrant conduction.

Aetiology

A re-entry circuit is the proposed underlying mechanism for PSVT. A re-entry circuit consists of two pathways that are connected at their upper and lower ends, providing an uninterrupted circuit for impulses conduction.

In AVNRT (atrioventricular nodal re-entrant tachycardia), a micro-re-entry circuit involving the two pathways (α and β) in the AV junction is implicated (Figs 4.17A and B). A supraventricular impulse travels slowly down the one pathway in the AV node towards the ventricles (a), but while in the way to ventricles, it is rapidly conducted back to atria through the second pathway within AV node (b). In this way atria and ventricles are depolarised almost simultaneously.

A vicious circle is set up that perpetuates and sustains the tachycardia (c). It is the commonest form of PSVT.

AVNRT is the most common type of narrow QRS complex tachycardia.

A

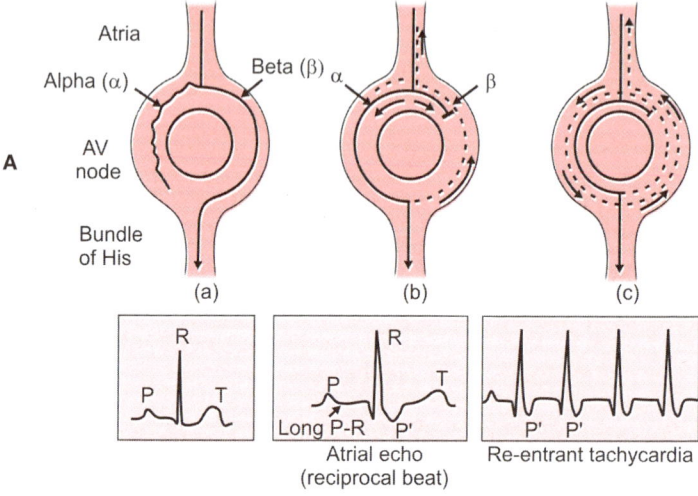

(a)   (b)   (c)

Atrial echo
(reciprocal beat)

Re-entrant tachycardia

B

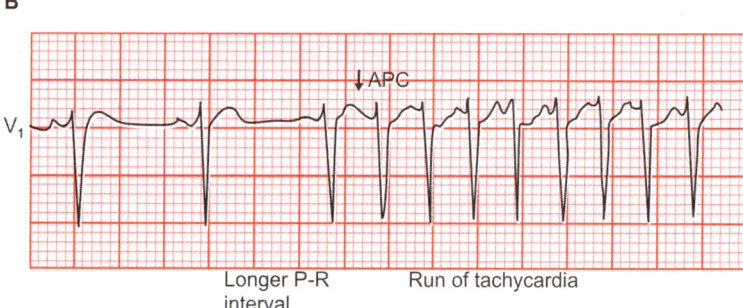

Longer P-R interval   Run of tachycardia

Figs 4.17A and B: A Mechanisms of AV nodal re-entry and re-entrant tachycardia. The atria, AV node and His bundle are diagrammatically shown. The AV node is longitudinally split into two different functional pathways, alpha (α) and beta (β). (a) During sinus rhythm, the impulse passes down the beta (fast) pathway to produce normal P-R interval. Conduction through alpha pathway cannot pass down due to refractoriness of the bundle of His as shown. (b) With a premature atrial beat, block occurs in fast beta pathway (indicated by a bar), hence, it passes down slowly through alpha pathway to the ventricles(long P-R interval). It gets retrogradely conducted to atria again (dotted line) to produce an atrial echo (P', reciprocal beat). See the diagram below where inverted P' wave follows QRS. This has occurred after long P-R interval which is pre-requisite for retrograde conduction. (c) When atrial premature beat is able to sustain circus movements through alpha and beta pathways, sustained AVNRT will result. The initiating event remains same, i.e. long P-R interval; (B) The ECG strip demonstrates a long P-R interval ($\downarrow$) of the atrial ectopic beat that initiates the tachycardia after which P wave is burried within QRS

The ECG characteristics of AVNRT (Fig. 4.18)

1. *Initiation and termination of tachycardia.* An atrial premature complex/beat (APC/APB) with a prolonged P-R interval initiates the tachycardia (Fig. 4.17B). The abrupt termination occurs with retrograde P wave, followed by period of asystole or bradycardia.
2. *The P waves are inverted* in leads II, III and aVF.
3. *The initiating P wave of an APC* is followed by a QRS complex, but subsequent beats/complexes reveal either a QRS complex followed by an inverted P' wave or a QRS complex with an embedded P' wave (P wave is not visible).
4. *The QRS complexes* are narrow and regular.
5. *The heart rate* (both atrial and ventricular rates) is > 100 bpm. The conduction ratio is 1:1, i.e. there is one P' wave for each QRS.
6. *There is ST segment depression and T wave inversion* during tachycardia (an associated change due to tachycardia) which reverts to normal after restoration of normal sinus rhythm.

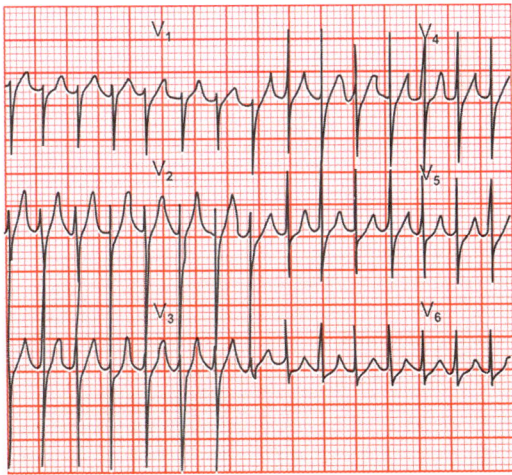

Fig. 4.18: Narrow QRS complex tachycardia—paroxysmal supraventricular tachycardia. The ECG (precordial leads V_1–V_6) shows heart rate of 187/min. The P waves are not visible because each P is superimposed on the preceding T wave making it a peaked T wave (normal T wave has rounded but not peaked top). Note: The initial initiating event is not recorded in the ECG, which is presumed to be an APC with prolonged P-R interval

Clinical Tips to PSVT

1. If the abnormal P' wave of the initiating APC is the same as the subsequent P waves of tachycardia; then it is an automatic paroxysmal atrial tachycardia.
2. If P-R interval of an APC initiating tachycardia is long, then it is AVNRT. If the APC initiating tachycardia is not seen (a common situation), in such a situation, the narrow QRS complexes with embedded P waves suggest AVNRT (Fig. 4.18).

VENTRICULAR ARRHYTHMIAS/DYSARRHYTHMIAS

When the pace of the heart is controlled by the ventricles, it is called *ventricular rhythm*. The ventricular rhythm is always abnormal and a slow rhythm.

Ventricular Ectopics/Extrasystole/Premature Complex

A premature discharge or an impulse originating from an ectopic focus within the ventricle is called *ventricular ectopic or ventricular premature complex* (VPC). It arises in the diastolic period of preceding sinus cycle, is recorded earlier than expected sinus beat.

Causes

The causes are given in Box 3

BOX 3: CAUSES OF VENTRICULAR PREMATURE COMPLEXES	
Common	*Uncommon*
• Physiological—no evidence of heart disease	• Alcohol intake
• Stress, anxiety, excessive tea and coffee intake	• Pericardial disease
• Coronary artery disease	• Cor pulmonale
• Acute myocardial infarction	• Following cardiac surgery or catheterisation
• Cardiomyopathies and myocarditis	• Metabolic disorder
• Valvular heart disease	• Congenital cardiac disease
• Digitalis induced	
• Hypertensive heart disease	• Poisoning, bites, etc.
• Electrolyte disturbance, e.g. hypokalemia	

The ECG characteristics (Figs 4.19A and B)

1. A VPC being premature occurs earlier than the expected sinus beat, hence, disturbs the sinus rhythm with the result, the R-R interval becomes irregular.
2. *The QRS morphology:* The QRS complex of a VPC is wider and bizarre because a VPC originates from the ectopic focus in a ventricle and then spreads abnormally through the ventricles.

Wide QRS > 0.14 sec is a characteristic feature of VPC.

3. *The relationship of P wave to QRS:* It varies because sinus discharge produces P wave and ventricular ectopic focus produces QRS. The P wave is embedded usually within QRS, hence P is not visible, but it can precede the wide QRS with a short P-R interval called an *end-diastolic VPC* or an inverted P wave may follow the wide QRS.
4. *Pre-ectopic interval:* The interval between a sinus beat and a VPC is called *pre-ectopic or coupling interval*, is fixed for all unifocal VPCs, but varies if VPCs are multifocal.

The pre-ectopic interval is shorter than post-ectopic (compensatory pause) interval.

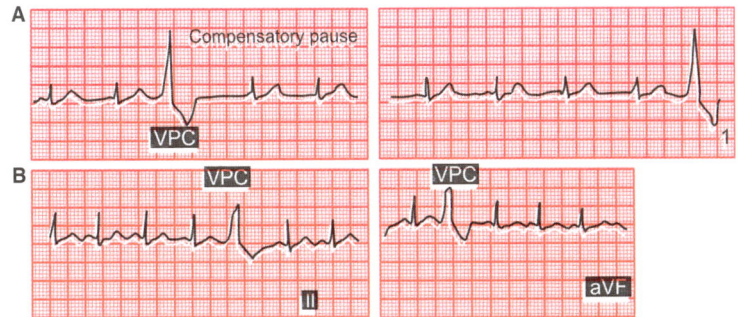

Figs 4.19A and B: Ventricular premature complexes (VPC labelled). (A) The complexes have no visible P waves (P is embedded within QRS), wide QRS > 0.14 sec with ST depression and T wave inversion; (B) Each VPC seen in leads II and aVF has a wide slurred QRS (> 0.14 sec) and depressed ST segment and inverted T wave. The P wave is embedded at the top of slurred R wave

5. *The compensatory pause:* A long interval that immediately follows the VPC and ends before next sinus beat is called *compensatory pause*. It is longer than pre-ectopic interval except in end-diastolic VPCs.

> ☞ *A compensatory pause (long post-ectopic interval) follows all premature complexes including VPCs (e.g. it follows the APC and AV nodal ectopics).*

6. *The ST-T change:* The VPC shows ST segment depression and T wave inversion as an associated change. This is not due to ventricular ischaemia.

How to Recognise a VPC?

Look at the rhythm strip carefully and pick up a complex which appears wider and bizarre. Now analyse the complex as follows:

- Is the QRS wider (> 0.14 sec)?
- Is the interval between the sinus beat and the VPC (pre-ectopic interval) is shorter than postectopic interval (interval between the VPC and next sinus beat)?
- Is a compensatory pause present after the complex?
- Does the complex show ST segment depression and T wave inversion?
- If all these characteristics are present then the complex is a VPC.

Types of VPCs

1. *An interpolated VPC:* A VPC sandwitched between the two sinus beats is called an interpolated VPC (Fig. 4.20).
2. *VPC with R on T phenomenon:* If the VPC either falls or comes with closer to the T wave of the preceding sinus beat, then it is called a VPC with R on T phenomenon. These (Fig. 4.21) VPCs predispose to the development of ventricular tachycardia or ventricular fibrillation, hence, called *pre-malignant VPCs.*
3. *Unifocal and multifocal VPCs:* The VPCs having similar shape in the same lead are called *unifocal VPCs* (Figs 4.22A and B)

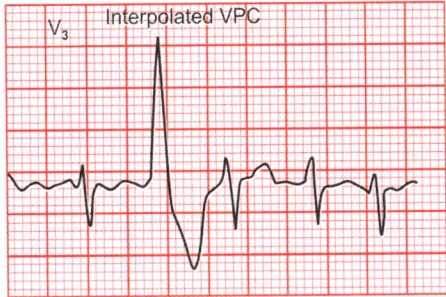

Fig. 4.20: Interpolated VPCs. The lead V$_3$ shows a VPC whose pre-ectopic and post-ectopic interval is equal (i.e. it is sandwiched between two sinus beats). There is no compensatory pause. It is an interpolated VPC

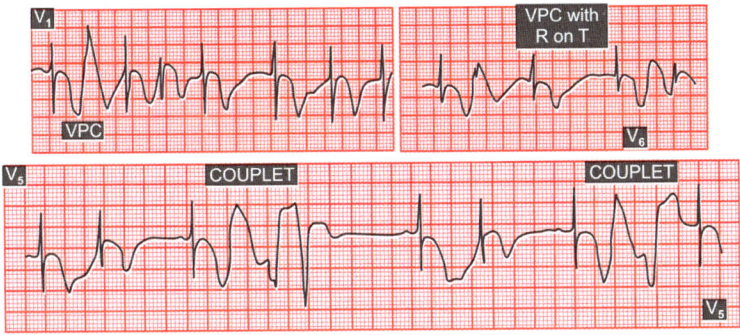

Fig. 4.21: Ventricular premature complexes (VPCs) with R on T phenomenon. The upper strip (leads V$_1$ and V$_6$) shows VPCs whose R wave is falling on the inverted T wave of sinus beat. There is ST segment depression with deep symmetric T wave inversion probably due to subendocardial ischaemia—the cause of VPCs. The lower strip (lead V$_5$) shows three sinus complexes followed by a ventricular couplet showing R and T phenomenon (the R wave of first VPC falls on the T of sinus beat and that of second VPC falls on the T of first VPC) The same process is repeated at the end of the strip

if shape of VPCs is different in the same lead, then they are called *multifocal VPCs* (Fig. 4.22B).

4. *Ventricular couplet:* The two VPCs in a row or a pair of VPCs is called a *ventricular couplet* (Figs 4.21 and 4.23).

5. *Ventricular bigeminy and trigeminy:* When a normal sinus beat alternates with a VPC in a regular fashion, it is called *ventricular bigeminy* (Fig. 4.24). A common cause of its

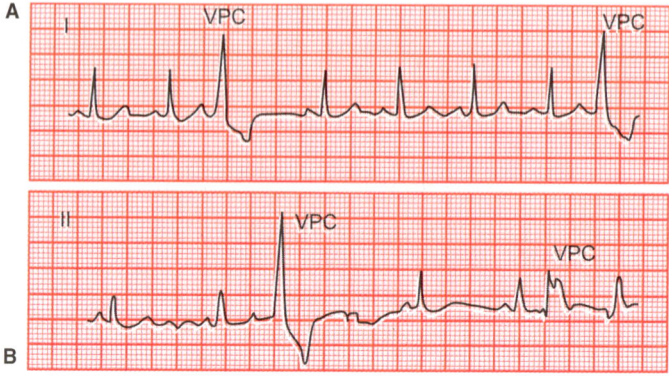

Figs 4.22A and B: Unifocal or monomorphic VPCs. (A) Upper strip (lead I) shows VPCs (labelled) with QRS complex having similar shape and direction (upright complex); (B) Lead II shows multifocal VPCs (labelled)

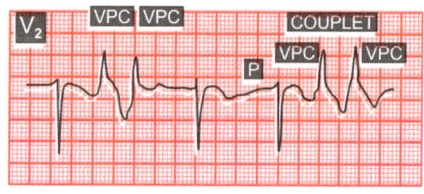

Fig. 4.23: Ventricular couplets (two in number). The lead V_2 shows a sinus beat followed by a couplet. The second couplet is seen at the end

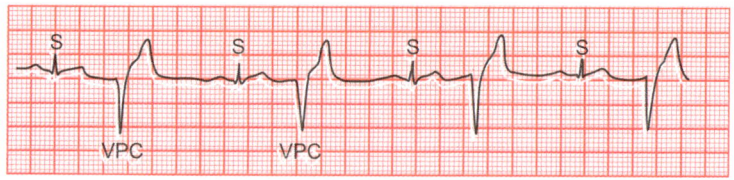

Fig. 4.24: Ventricular bigeminy. The lead II shows a sinus beat (S) alternating with a VPC (labelled) in a rhythmic fashion called bigeminy rhythm

digitalis. The interval between the sinus beat and the VPC is fixed called *fixed coupling (pre-ectopic) interval of unifocal VPCs.*

When two normal sinus beats are followed by a VPC and this pattern is repeated in a rhythmic fashion, then it is called ventricular trigeminy (Fig. 4.25).

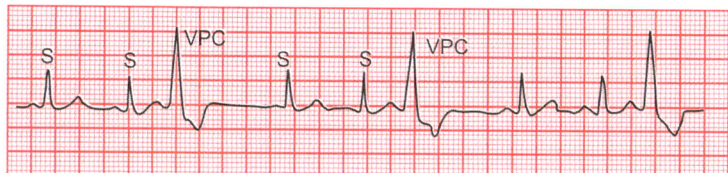

Fig. 4.25: Ventricular trigeminy. A VPC comes after two sinus complexes (S) in a rhythmic fashion called *trigeminus rhythm*

Clinical significance

They are among the most common arrhythmias that occur in patients with or without heart disease. Although isolated VPCs, may occur occasionally in normal persons without heart disease, but their presence should always be viewed with suspicion.

The VPCs are always significant if associated with heart ailment. Multifocal or polymorphic VPCs, or ventricular complex with R on T phenomenon are always abnormal and indicate a serious myocardial disease and require immediate attention and treatment. Unifocal or monomorphic VPCs are indicative of heart disease if:
- They occur frequently (> 10/min)
- They show R on T phenomenon
- They occur in a setting of heart disease
- They occur in patients above 40 years
- They are precipitated by exercise.

Remember

Ventricular couplets and VPCs with R on T phenomenon are harbingers of ventricular tachycardia and ventricular fibrillation.

Idioventricular Rhythm/Accelerated Idioventricular Rhythm

The intrinsic rhythm of the ventricles is called *an idioventricular rhythm.* Normally, this rhythm is suppressed by higher pacemakers (SA and AV node), appears only when the SA nodal and AV nodal pacemakers are dysfunctional.

It is defined as a slow escape rhythm originating from the ventricle at a rate of 15–40 bpm. When it accelerates its rate beyond 45 bpm but less than 100 bpm (usually 70–80 bpm) then it is called an *accelerated idioventricular rhythm.*

Causes

The causes are given in Box 4

BOX 4: CAUSES OF IDIOVENTRICULAR RHYTHM	
• Acute MI	• Cardiomyopathies
• Myocarditis	• Drugs (e.g. digoxin)
• Trauma	• Dying heart
• Following reperfusion or DC shock	• Complete heart block

The ECG characteristics (Fig. 4.26)

1. The ventricular rate (heart rate) is regular.
2. The ventricular rate is slow between 15 and 45 bpm.
3. The QRS complexes are wide and bizarre and all look alike.
4. The P waves may or may not be present. The absence of P indicates that the higher pacemaker, e.g. SA node is not firing.

The presence of P indicates presence of two pacemakers; one in the atrium and other in the ventricles as occurs in complete heart block. These two pacemakers fire independently, hence, P wave have no fixed relation to QRS.

In complete heart block, the ventricular rhythm is idioventricular and is independent of normal sinus rhythm (there is dual rhythm in complete heart block).

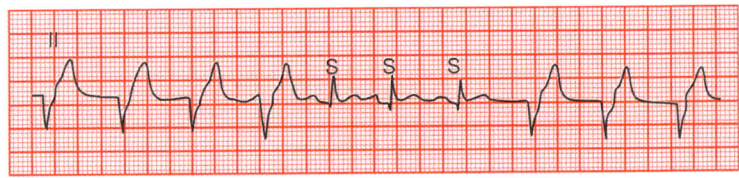

Fig. 4.26: Accelerated idioventricular rhythm. The lead II shows initial four wide QRS complexes without preceding P wave occurring at a rate of 93/min, regularly indicating an accelerated idioventricular rhythm which gets terminated and followed by next 3 normal QRS complexes (S). At the end of the strip, an accelerated idioventricular rhythm reappears at the same rate

Ventricular Tachycardia (VT)

Definition

Ventricular tachycardia is defined as a series of three or more consecutive ventricular ectopics or premature complexes

(VPCs) which are recorded in a rapid succession. It is either due to enhanced automaticity of a ventricular ectopic focus (rare) or due to re-entry within the ventricular myocardium (common).

Causes

The causes are given in Box 5

BOX 5: CAUSES OF VENTRICULAR TACHYCARDIA	
• Acute myocardial infarction or ischaemia	• Hypokalaemia
• Cardiomyopathies	• Drug induced (e.g. digitalis and other proarrhythmics)
• Myocarditis • Reperfusion • Ventricular aneurysm	• Mechanically induced by a pacing catheter or flow directed pulmonary artery catheter or pacemaker induced (DDD pacemaker)
• Idiopathic arrhythmogenic right ventricular dysplasia	• Idiopathic (unknown cause)

The ECG characteristics (Figs 4.27 and 4.28)

1. The QRS complexes characteristics:
   - They are wide and bizarre
   - The QRS duration is > 0.14 sec
   - The QRS complexes may look alike (monomorphic) or may have different shapes (polymorphic), may occur in one direction or alternately in both the directions (bidirectional).

2. The ventricular rate is >100 bpm, can be regular or slightly irregular. Ventricular rate > 200 bpm is unusual for VT.

3. The superior left axis deviation ($-90°$ to $-180°$) with positive deflection in leads I and aVR and negative deflection in lead III.

4. *A run of ventricular ectopics:* There are at least three successive ventricular ectopics in a row.

5. *AV dissociation:* There is AV dissociation, i.e. the P waves have no relation to QRS.

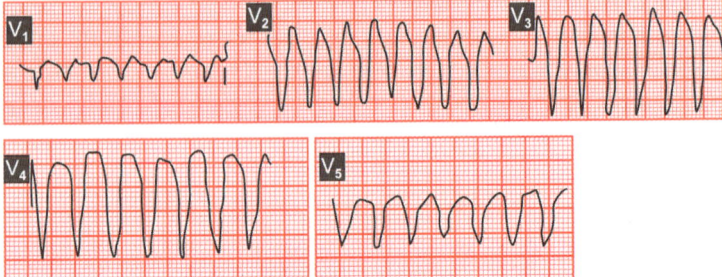

Fig. 4.27: Ventricular tachycardia. The ECG (V_1–V_5) shows (i) Broad (wide) QRS complex (0.14 sec) tachycardia at a rate of 187/min; (ii) Concordant pattern (all complexes are negative from (V_1–V_5)

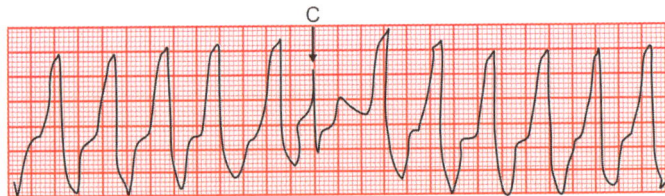

Fig. 4.28A: Ventricular tachycardia (VT). (i) There is a wide QRS complex tachycardia (QRS > 0.14 sec); (ii) There is single narrow complex in the centre called *capture beat* (labelled as C), indicates that a supraventricular beat has captured the ventricles without interrupting tachycardia—a characteristic feature of VT

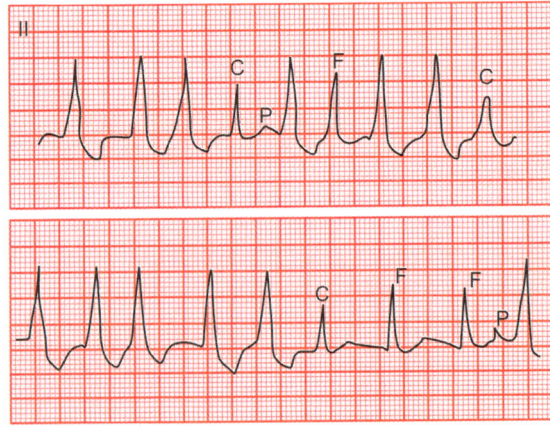

Fig. 4.28B: Ventricular tachycardia (VT). The lead II (continuous) shows wide QRS complex (> 0.14 sec) tachycardia at a rate of > 150/min which is irregular at times. The P waves (two P are labelled) do not have any relation to QRS, indicate AV dissociation. The fusion beats—a characteristic of VT, are seen (labelled as F), display variable degree of fusion. Few capture beats (C) are also seen—a characteristic feature of VT

6. *Fusion beats and capture beats:* These are characteristic features of VT.
   a. *A capture beat* is a normal conducted sinus beat within the run of VT, indicates that a sinus impulse has captured the ventricle. It is diagnostic of VT.
   b. *A fusion complex* (a partial capture) is produced by activation of the ventricles both by sinus and ectopic beats, hence, it is a blend complex whose configuration is intermediate between the normal sinus beat and ventricular ectopic.

The presence of capture beat (s) or fusion beat (s) within the run of VT is diagnostic of VT, occurs as a result of AV dissociation.

7. *Concordant pattern of QRS in precordial leads:* The concordant pattern in chest leads (V_1–V_6) means that the QRS complexes are either upright or downwards in all the leads. It is a pattern characteristic of VT.
8. *Ventricular ectopic with R on T phenomenon* may be seen triggering the VT.
9. *Initiation and termination:* The VPC (a critically late VPC or VPC with R on T phenomenon) initiates the VT spontaneously. Nonsustained VT terminates spontaneously, while sustained VT require termination because of haemodynamic consequence.

Diagnostic clues to VT
• A run (> 3 VPCs) of wide QRS (> 0.14 sec) complex tachycardia
• Ventricular rate > 100/min
• The superior axis ≥140° (R in leads I and aVR, S in III)
• Concordant pattern in precordial leads
• AV dissociation—a characteristic feature
• Presence of fusion complexes and capture beats within a run of VT

Differentiation of VT from SVT with aberration (Box 6)

Types of VT

1. *Sustained vs nonsustained:* VT lasting more than 30 seconds is called sustained and if remains for < 30 secs, then it is called nonsustained (Fig. 4.29).

BOX 6: DIFFERENTIATING WIDE QRS TACHYCARDIA

Feature	Supraventricular tachycardia (SVT) with aberration (Fig. 4.28C)	Ventricular tachycardia (VT)
1. P wave	A premature P may precede QRS	Not preceded by P wave
2. QRS morphology	rSR' in V_1 and RS with wide S in V_6	Slurred R, RR' or QR in V_1 or rS or qR in V_6
3. QRS duration	> 0.14 sec	< 0.14 sec
4. R-R interval	Regular	Regular, can be irregular
5. Axis	Right or left	Left and superior
6. QRS pattern	Nonconcordant	Concordant
7. AV dissociation	Not seen	Seen
8. Fusion and capture beats	Absent	Present—a characteristic feature

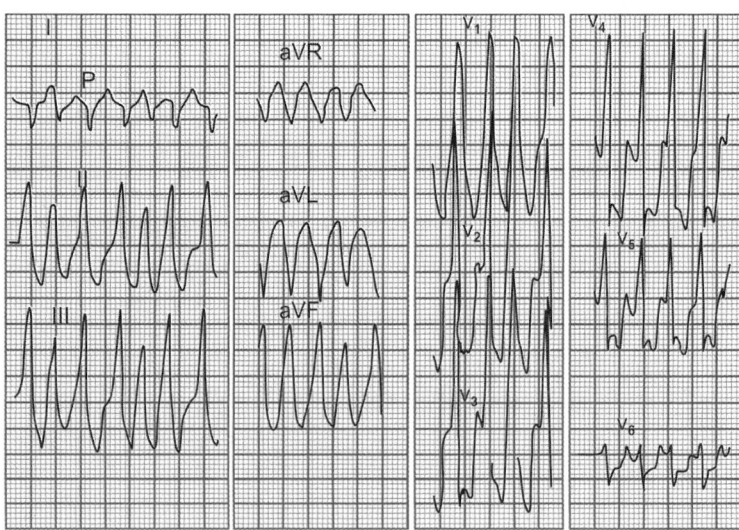

Fig. 4.28C: Supraventricular tachycardia with aberrant conduction. There is right axis deviation with wide QRS complexes (> 0.14 sec). There is right bundle branch block pattern in V_1 and RS complexes with wide S in V_6. The QRS complexes are preceded by P waves as seen in lead I (labelled). There are neither fusion nor capture beats. All these features suggest SVT with aberrant conduction

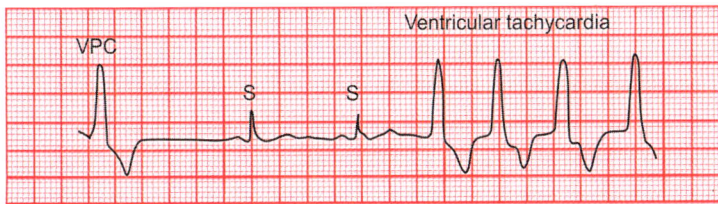

Fg. 4.29: Nonsustained self-terminating VT. There are four wide QRS complexes (> 0.14 sec) constituting nonsustained VT following normal two QRS complexes (S) indicating sinus rhythm. The heart rate is > 100/min. The first QRS is a VPC

2. *Monomorphic vs polymorphic:* If all the QRS complexes in a run of VT look alike, then, it is monomorphic and if they differ in configuration in the same lead, then it is polymorphic VT.

Torsades de Pointes (TdP)

It is a variant of polymorphic ventricular tachycardia is which QRS complexes of varying amplitudes appear to twist around the baseline, hence, its name torsades de pointes (e.g. twisting of pointes). It is characteristically seen after prolonged Q-T interval. It is often self-limiting but can degenerate into ventricular fibrillation.

Causes

1. Class I antiarrhythmics.
2. Hypokalaemia, hypocalcaemia and hypomagnesaemia.
3. Psychotropic drugs (e.g. phenothiazines, antidepressants, antihistaminics, pentamidine and some antimalarials).
4. Acute myocardial infarction or Prinzmetal's angina.
5. Weight reducing liquid protein diets and starvation.
6. Congenital prolonged Q-T syndrome.
7. Acquired prolonged Q-T due to any cause.
8. CNS lesions.
9. Mitral valve prolapse.

The ECG characteristics (Fig. 4.30)

1. The polarity of QRS complexes alternates around the baseline. The QRS complexes tend to be bizarre, multiform and their axis undulates for a short period of few seconds, hence, for a moment complexes are directed upwards and then immediately downwards.

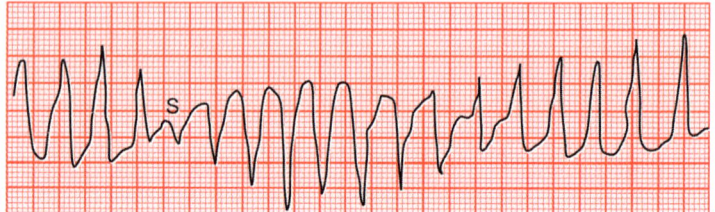

Fig. 4.30: Torsades de pointes. The rhythm strip shows broad complex polymorphic ventricular tachycardia in which QRS complexes are twisting along the baseline. This follows a sinus beat with prolonged Q-T interval which initiates it (S)

2. It is usually initiated by a VPC with prolonged QTc interval or a VPC with R on T phenomenon.
3. The amplitude of QRS complexes may show waxing and waning.
4. The ventricular rate is extremely rapid (200–250 bpm).

Ventricular Fibrillation (Fig. 4.31)

Ventricular fibrillation is a catastrophic dysarrhythmia characterised by disorganised electrical activity of the heart. In the absence of ECG monitoring, it is difficult to distinguish it from ventricular asystole.

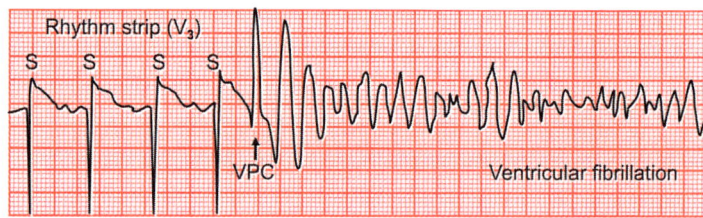

Fig. 4.31: Ventricular fibrillation (VF). Rhythm strips (V₃) shows 4 initial beats as sinus beat (S) with ST elevation indicating ST elevation myocardial infarction (STEMI). This is followed by an ventricular ectopic beat (VPC↑) that initiates an episode of ventricular fibrillation in which there is no identifiable waveform. The baseline during VF is undulating due to bizarre complexes that vary in size and shape

Causes

- Myocardial ischaemia or infarction
- Cardiomyopathy
- Electrolyte abnormalities

- Drug toxicity
- Accidental electric shock
- Failure to synchronise DC shock.

ECG characteristics

- No waveform is identifiable
- Bizaree complexes of varying size and shape undulate the baseline.

Ventricular Asystole

It is defined as complete absence of electrical activity of the heart. Asystole, also called cardiac standstill, represents the terminal cardiac events (dyeing heart) and cannot be distinguished from ventricular fibrillation without ECG monitoring.

Causes

1. Protracted episodes of VF.
2. Failure of pacemaker activity of the heart due to any cause such as drugs, acute MI and so forth.
3. A terminal event in all acute catastrophic cardiovascular conditions.

The ECG characteristics (Fig. 4.32)

- No ECG waveforms are identifiable.
- The baseline appears wavy or flat as a straight line.

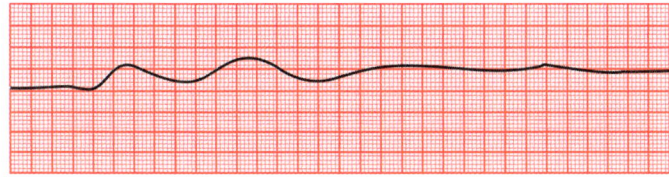

Fig. 4.32: Ventricular asystole. The baseline is more or less straight without any waveform

Caution

Before labelling it as asystole, a different lead may be recorded to show baseline straight. The electric main supply or power connections must be checked.

AMBULATORY (HOLTER) ELECTROCARDIOGRAPHY

Continuous ambulatory electrocardiographic recording (Holter monitoring) is a method by which ECG is recorded continuously for specified period of time while the patient is carrying out his/her normal activities. The test can be done on an out-patient basis.

Indications

1. *Detection of an arrhythmia:* The widely accepted indication of Holter monitoring is to detect arrhythmia/dysarrhythmia and to correlate it with patient's symptoms, e.g. palpitation, syncope, fatigue and dyspnoea.
2. *Detection of myocardial ischaemia or coronary artery spasm:* Silent or painful episodes of myocardial ischaemia during day-time activities can be detected and documented by 24 hour Holter monitoring.

   Holter monitoring is also useful in detecting ST segment elevation in patients with Prinzmetal's angina because ST segment elevation does not occur during stress testing, hence, Holter monitoring is superior diagnostic parameter for this condition than stress testing.

Lead system used (Fig. 4.33)

Usually, two leads (V_1 and V_2) are recorded for which 5 electrodes are needed in bipolar lead system.

The electrodes are placed as depicted in Fig. 4.33.

The patient wears monitoring electrodes attached to a portable device that records the cardiac rhythm continuously on the tape over a period of 12, 24, or 48 hours. The patient continues to perform his/her normal daily activities while the test is in progress and patient is asked to record significant events and associated symptoms in a diary (including time). The significant events on the recording system can be recorded by event recorder. The patient can wear the recorder continuously, activating it when symptomatic. At the completion of the test, the stored rhythm is scanned to detect arrhythmia, heart blocks or ST segment change. Events recorded in the diary (including associated symptoms) are correlated with the cardiac rhythm recorded on the Holter tracing at that time. Few tracings from Holter monitoring are depicted in Fig. 4.34.

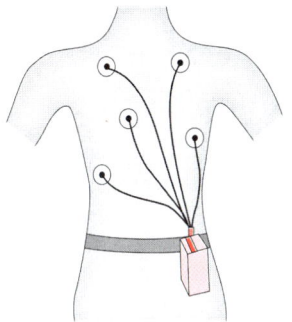

Fig. 4.33: Holter monitoring. Electrodes placed on the body surface for continuous recording of ECG over a period of hours to days

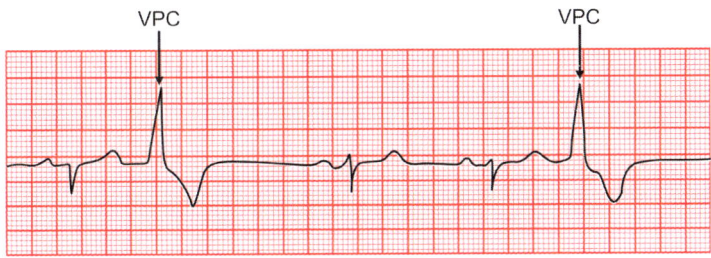

Holter monitor tracing showing unifocal VPCs (↓)

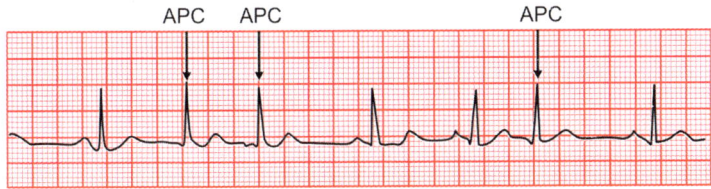

Holter monitor tracing showing atrial premature complexes (APCs)

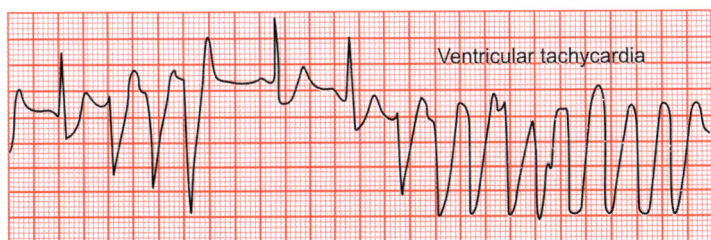

Holter monitor tracing showing intermittent wide QRS complex tachycardia

Fig. 4.34: Tracing from Holter monitoring

5

Abnormalities of P Waves, QRS Complexes and T Waves

- Abnormalities of P wave
- Abnormalities of QRS complexes
- Abnormalities of T wave
- Abnormalities of ST segment and T wave

While interpreting ECG, first of all look at the rhythm and heart rate. Now look at the followings:

- What is direction of cardiac axis (read chapter 1)?
- Is there any electrical rotation of heart (read chapter 1)?
- Look at the P wave. Is there any abnormality of P wave?
- Look at the P-R interval. Calculate it (normal or abnormal).
- Look at the QRS complexes. Note any abnormality of Q wave and R wave. Measure the duration of QRS complex.
- Now look at the ST segment. Is the ST segment isoelectric, depressed below the baseline or raised above the baseline?

ABNORMALITIES OF THE P WAVE

The P wave is produced by synchronized depolarization of both atria, hence, its abnormalities reflect atrial hypertrophy. The P wave abnormalities occur either in its amplitude (tall P wave more than normal) or in its width/duration (wide P wave more than normal).

ATRIAL HYPERTROPHY

As we know, the P wave represents the atrial events, hence, atrial hypertrophy is reflected in the abnormalities of P wave.

Since the SA node is situated in the right atrium, therefore, right atrial activation is immediately followed by left atrial activation. The normal P wave is blend of both the activations. When one atrium, enlarges, the activation process is disturbed resulting in either increase in length or duration of P wave. The leads II and V_1 are best for abnormality of the P wave (Figs 5.1A and B) to be seen.

Left Atrial Hypertrophy

Normally, the P wave has two components, i.e. initial right atrial and terminal left atrial, both components form normal P wave. In left atrial hypertrophy, the terminal left atrial (LA) component becomes prominent leading to splitting of the P wave in which initial component is small and terminal is large called *P mitrale*. In standard leads (II, III and aVF), the P wave is seen as bifid P wave while in lead V_1 (Figs 5.1A) it is seen as biphasic P wave with wide and slurred terminal negative component. Sometimes, these two components may not be seen separately resulting in widening of P wave > 2.5 mm.

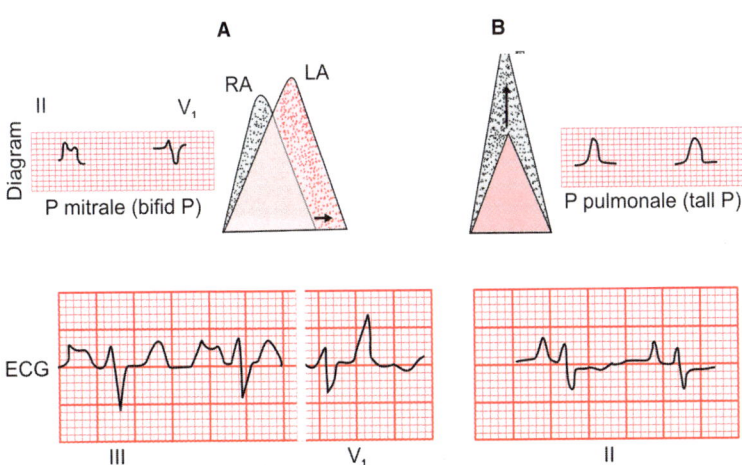

Figs 5.1A and B: Abnormalities of P wave. (A) Left atrial hypertrophy; (B) Right atrial hypertrophy

Causes

The causes are given in Box 1

BOX 1: CAUSES OF LEFT ATRIAL HYPERTROPHY
• Ventricular septal defect (VSD)
• Left sided valvular lesion, e.g. mitral stenosis/mitral regurgitation
• Aortic stenosis
• Systemic hypertension
• Cardiomyopathy
• Left atrial myxoma

The ECG characteristics (Fig. 5.2)

- Increase in width of P wave > 2.5 mm.
- Bifid P wave (P mitrale) in standard leads and biphasic P with widened slurred terminal component in lead V_1.

Remember

Wide or bifid P wave (P mitrale) indicates left atrial hypertrophy.

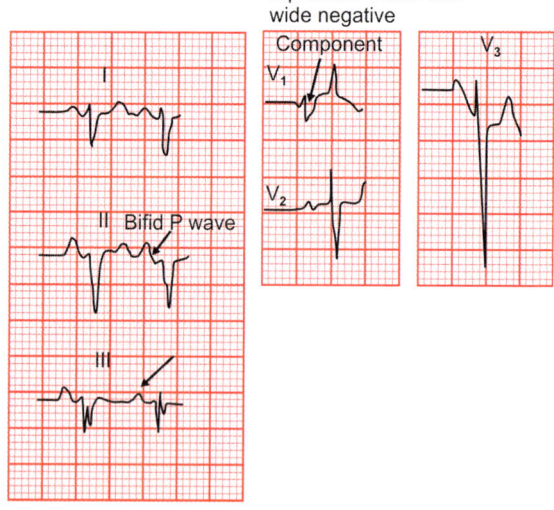

Fig. 5.2: Left atrial hypertrophy–P mitrale (bifid P wave in standard leads (I, II, III) indicated by arrows and biphasic P with widened terminal negative component in precordial leads (V_1–V_2) one of them is labelled and indicated by an arrow

Right Atrial Hypertrophy

Right atrial hypertrophy produces an increase in the muscle mass of atrium resulting in increase in height of P wave called *P pulmonale* (Fig. 5.3). The duration of P wave does not increase.

Causes

The causes are given in Box 2

BOX 2: CAUSES OF RIGHT ATRIAL HYPERTROPHY
• Atrial septal defect (ASD)
• Lutembacher syndrome
• Right-sided valvular lesion, e.g. tricuspid stenosis and tricuspid regurgitation
• Pulmonary stenosis
• Pulmonary hypertension
• Cor pulmonale
• Right atrial myxoma

The ECG characteristics (Fig. 5.3)

1. Increase in amplitude of P wave > 2.5 mm, best seen in leads II, III and aVF. In the lead V_1, the initial upward component of biphasic P is prominent and taller than terminal negative component. The negative component may become absent and resulting just in tall monophasic P wave.
2. The duration of P does not increase.

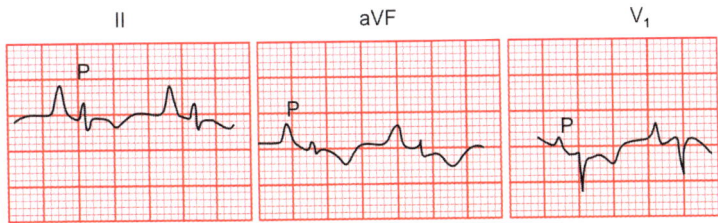

Fig. 5.3: The P wave is tall (> 2.5 mm) in leads II, aVF and V_1

Remember

The tall P wave > 2.5 mm in standard leads indicate right atrial hypertrophy.

Biatrial Hypertrophy

Biatrial hypertrophy results in an increase in the amplitude of P wave (> 2.5 mm) as well as width of P wave (> 2.5 mm) because both the components become prominent, hence, the lead V_1 the P waveis biphasic with accentuation of both initial upright and terminal negative deflections.

The ECG characteristics (Fig. 5.4)

1. Wide and notched P waves in standard leads.
2. Tall and wide biphasic P wave in lead V_1.

> *Remember*
>
> *The tall and wide P waves in standard leads indicate biatrial hypertrophy.*

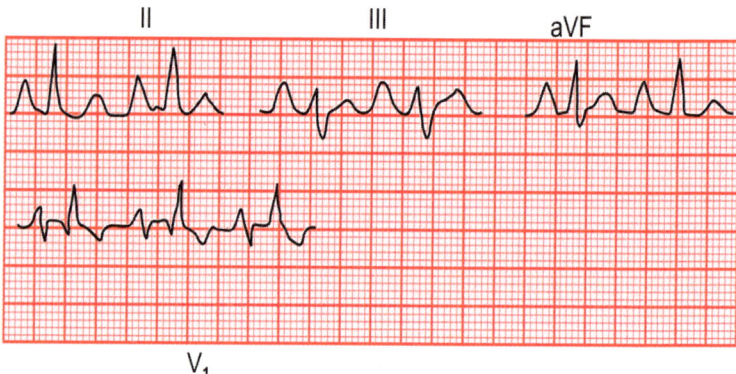

Fig. 5.4: Biatrial hypertrophy: P wave is wide and tall in leads II, III, and aVF (labelled). In V_1—the upward deflection is prominent as well as negative downward deflection (labelled)

THE ABNORMALITIES OF QRS COMPLEX

Characteristics of QRS Complex

- The QRS complex is < 0.12 sec normally in all the leads.
- The sum of QRS in leads V_1 and V_5 does not exceed 35 mm (except in young adults normally).
- Voltage of QRS complex is decreased in obese/thick chest individuals.

The abnormalities of QRS complex occur either in amplitude (height) or in duration (width).

- Low amplitude of QRS < 5 mm in standard leads called *low voltage, graph,* occurs in obesity, emphysema, myxoedema and pericardial effusion.
- Increase in voltage more than normal indicate ventricular hypertrophy (right or left).
- Increase in width of QRS occurs due to prolonged depolarisation either due to bundle branch block or an abnormal focus in the ventricle initiating ectopic beat(s) or tachycardia or idioventricular rhythm.

VENTRICULAR HYPERTROPHY

Ventricular hypertrophy is a pathophysiologic consequence of sufficient workload (volume or pressure) on the either ventricle. In fact, ventricle hypertrophies as a compromise to augment the ventricular contraction to overcome the overload.

Pathogenesis of ECG changes in ventricular hypertrophy (Figs 5.5A and B).

1. *Increase in amplitude or voltage of QRS:* In ventricular hypertrophy, the height of QRS (especially R wave) is increased in the leads representing the ventricle, e.g. the leads V_5–V_6 in LVH and in lead V_1 and V_2 in RVH. This is due to altered geometric projection of electrical forces not an increase in muscle mass.
2. *Widening of QRS:* The QRS complex widens due to delayed conduction through the hypertrophied ventricle. The QRS interval does not exceed 0.12 sec. The ventricular activation time (VAT) is increased. These changes again are seen in the leads representing the ventricle.
3. *The ST depression:* The ST segment depression occurs in the leads representing the ventricle. This is due to relative myocardial ischaemia of hypertrophied ventricle.
4. *The T wave inversion:* T wave is inverted in the leads representing the ventricle. The T wave inversion is asymmetric.

For ventricular hypertrophy, leads V_1 and V_2 represent the right ventricle and leads V_5 and V_6 represent the left ventricle.

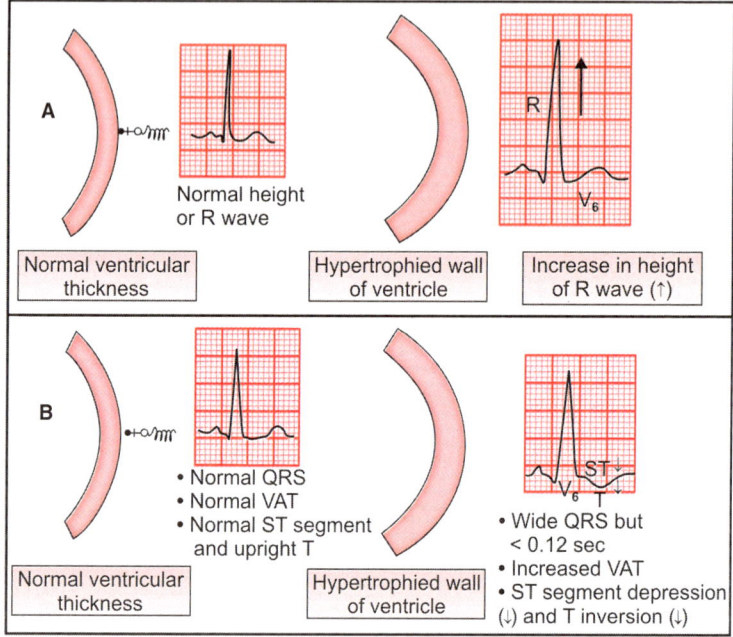

Figs 5.5A and B: Pathogenesis of ECG changes in a ventricular hypertrophy: (A) Height of R wave in normal and hypertrophied ventricle; (B) Conduction through normal versus hypertrophied ventricle and the ST-T changes in normal versus hypertrophied ventricle

Ventricular Strain

Ventricular strain in terms of electrocardiography represents more acute and reversible ST segment depression and T wave inversion which usually is not expected from the ventricular hypertrophy alone. The 'strain' probably reflects the expression of relative ventricular ischaemia.

> *Remember*
> - *If the above mention changes shown in Figs 5.5A and B. (increase in R wave and ST-T changes) occur in right-sided leads (V_1), they indicate RVH.*
> - *If these changes occur in left-sided precordial leads (V_5 or V_6), they indicate LVH.*
> - *If these changes occur in all the precordial leads (V_1–V_6) then they indicate biventricular hypertrophy.*

Left Ventricular Hypertrophy (LVH)

It refers to hypertrophy of free walls and apical regions of left ventricle as a result of overloading (systolic or diastolic) of the left ventricle.

Causes of LVH

1. *Systolic (pressure) overload*
   - Systemic hypertension
   - Aortic stenosis (valvular, subvalvular and supravalvular)
   - Coarctation of aorta
   - Hypertrophic cardiomyopathy
2. *Diastolic (volume) overload*
   - Aortic regurgitation
   - Mitral incompetence / regurgitation
   - Ventricular septal defect
   - Patent ductus arteriosus
   - Beri-Beri heart disease or other high cardiac output states.
3. *Myocardial diseases*
   - Coronary artery disease
   - Dilated cardiomyopathy

The electrocardiographic criteria (Figs 5.6 and 5.7)

1. *Abnormalities of QRS*

   i. *Increased amplitude of QRS:* The voltage criteria are given in Box 3.

   ii. Increased ventricular activation time in leads V_5–V_6 > 0.06 sec

   iii. Increased duration of QRS but less than 0.12 sec (usually between 0.10 and 0.12 sec).

   iv. Left axis deviation of QRS in frontal plane but less than −30°.

   v. Counterclockwise rotation of the heart resulting in shifting of transition zone to leads V_1 or V_2

2. *The ST-T changes:* There is ST segment depression and T wave inversion in leads V_3–V_6 in strain pattern (Fig. 5.7).

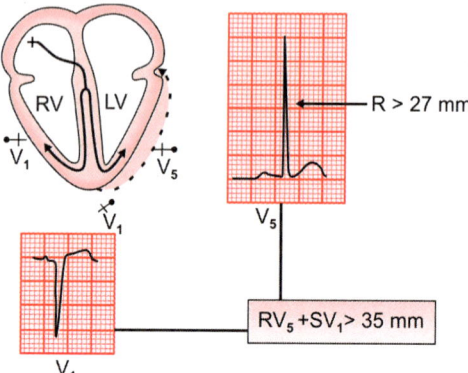

Fig. 5.6: Pathogenesis of big R (> 27 mm) and deep S. The increased left ventricular forces generated in LVH produces tall R in lead V_5 (shown) and deep S in lead V_1 (shown) and; the $RV_5 + SV_1$ is > 35 mm

☞ *LVH is characterised by height of R wave > 27 mm in V_5 or V_6, or $RV_5 + SV_1$, > 35 mm, with left axis deviation, horizontal heart and counterclockwise rotation.*
Tip: Always look for precordial leads V_5–V_6 for R wave; and V_1 or V_2 for S wave to diagnose LVH.

The left ventricular hypertrophy on ECG can be diagnosed by point scoring system described by Romhilt-Estes (Box 3).

BOX 3: ROMHILT-ESTES POINT SCORING SYSTEM	
1. Increase in QRS voltage	3 points
• R or S in limb lead > 20 mm	
• S in V_1 or $V_2 \geq 30$ mm	
• R in V_5 or $Y_6 \geq 30$ mm	
2. ST-T changes–without digitalis	3 points
with digitalis	1 point
3. Left axis deviation: 30° or more	2 points
4. QRS interval ≥ 0.09 sec	1 point
5. VAT in V_5 or $V_6 \geq 0.05$ sec	1 point
6. Left atrial abnormality	3 points

Note: Left ventricular hypertrophy is considered to be present if the total score is > 5 points, and probably present if the score is 4 points (Fig. 5.7).

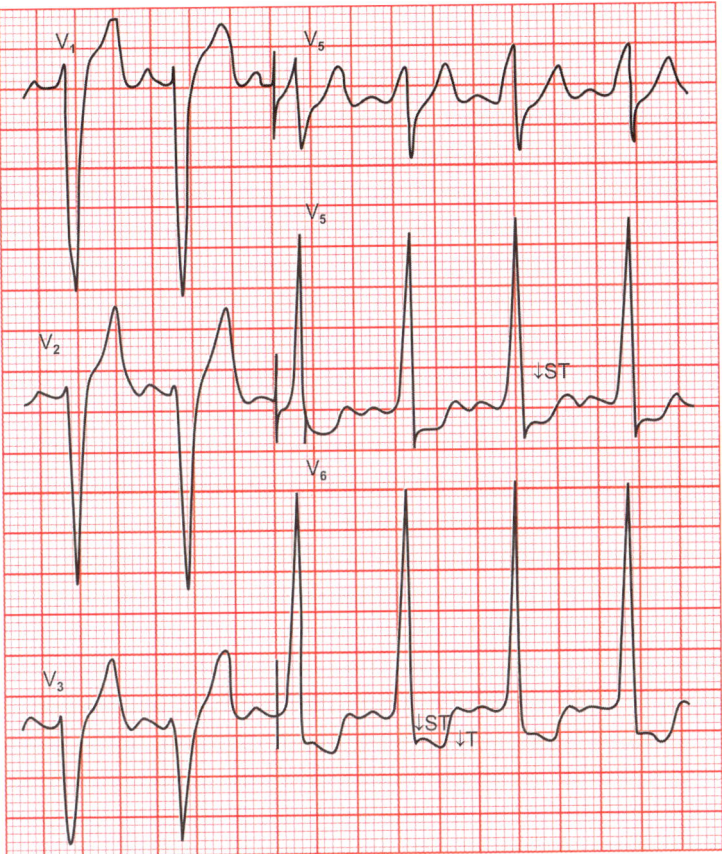

Fig. 5.7: Left ventricular hypertrophy with strain. The ECG (V_1–V_6) shows R wave in V_5 is 25 mm and $RV_5 + SV_1 = 25 + 25 = 50$ mm indicating LVH. There is significant ST depression ($\downarrow$) and T wave inversion (labelled) in V_5–V_6 indicating strain pattern

Right Ventricular Hypertrophy (RVH)

It refers to hypertrophy of the free walls of right ventricle along with paraseptal region or parabasal region or both.

Causes of RVH

1. Pulmonary hypertension either primary or secondary to mitral valve disease especially mitral stenosis.
2. Chronic cor pulmonale.

3. Congenital heart disease, e.g. pulmonary stenosis, tetralogy of Fallot, Eisenmenger's syndrome.
4. Associated with LVH.
5. Acute pulmonary thromboembolism.
6. Left to right shunts, e.g. ASD and VSD.
7. Cardiomyopathy (rare).

The electrocardiography criteria (Figs 5.8 and 5.9)

When right ventricular hypertrophy occurs, then left ventricular dominance is blunted by the augmented forces generated from the right ventricle. The QRS complex (i.e. R wave) in V_1 becomes more positive than normal and this R wave may become equal to S wave. In lead V_6, the QRS becomes blunted and balanced by right ventricle with the result a prominent deep S wave appears in V_5 and V_6 which is more than normal S wave in these leads. Therefore, ECG characteristics of right ventricular hypertrophy will be:

- The height of R wave is more than or equal to S wave in V_1 ($R \geq S$).
- VAT in lead V_1 is increased > 0.03.
- The R wave is greater than 7 mm in lead V_1 and greater than 5 mm in lead aVR.

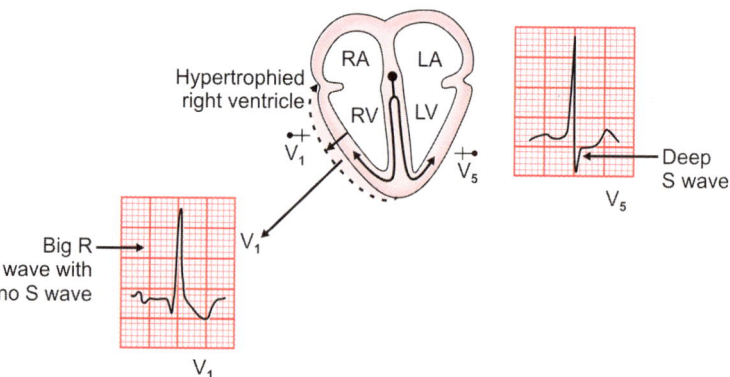

Fig. 5.8: Right ventricular hypertrophy (RVH). The increased right ventricular forces generated (←) produce big R in V_1 and corresponding deep and wide S in V_5–V_6

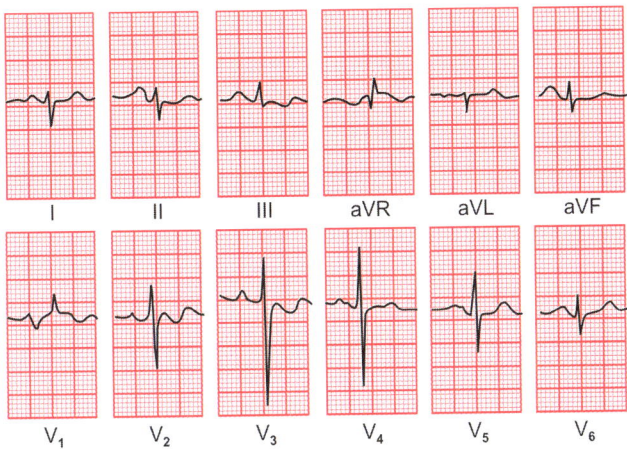

Fig. 5.9: Right ventricular and left atrial hypertrophy. The ECG shows (i) *Left atrial hypertrophy*. There is wide P wave (> 2.5 mm in leads II, III and aVF and a biphasic P wave with deep prominent negative component in V_1; (ii) *Right ventricular hypertrophy (RVH)*. There is a tall R wave with no S wave in V_1 with persistence of deep and wide S waves in V_5–V_6. There is associated right axis deviation and vertical heart position and clockwise rotation

- There is persistence of deep S wave (≥ 7 mm) in leads V_5 and V_6.
- *The ST-T changes:* There is ST segment depression and T wave inversion in leads V_1 and V_2.
- Right axis deviation
- Vertical heart position
- Clockwise rotation.

Remember

Always look at lead V_1 for large R wave in RVH.

Causes of increased height of R wave in V_1

- Normal in infants and children.
- Persistent juvenile pattern.
- Posterior wall infarction.
- Right bundle branch block.
- Mirror image dextrocardia.
- WPW syndrome (left side Kent bundle).

Biventricular Hypertrophy

Sometime, both ventricles of the heart become hypertrophied.

Causes

1. Dilated cardiomyopathy.
2. Congenital heart disease, e.g. Eisenmenger's syndrome.
3. Congestive heart failure with valvular lesions.
4. High cardiac output failure or state.

The electrocardiographic criteria

In biventricular hypertrophy, the forces from both the ventricles are increased, but the forces of left ventricular hypertrophy (LVH) dominate over right ventricular forces (a normal phenomenon), hence, the characteristic pattern of LVH will be usually seen in left precordial leads (V_5–V_6) and the right ventricular hypertrophy is detected only by right axis deviation.

Sometimes, the right ventricular hypertrophy also dominates and becomes equal to left ventricular hypertrophy, in such a situation, the right ventricular forces either blunt or cancel the left ventricular forces with the result a balanced state of forces is produced in which the right ventricular leads (V_1 and V_2) register RVH (R ≥ S wave or R : S > 1) while left ventricular leads (V_5 and V_6) register LVH. This result in Katz-Wachtel phenomenon where the transition zone remains at normal position (V_3 or V_4) but records a tall R wave and S wave which are equal (tall R = tall S).

In advance RVH, increasing right ventricular forces cancel the some of the left ventricular forces; in that situation, the voltage criteria of LVH may not be evident, hence, the LVH is detected by either left axis deviation or by other associated criteria. The criteria of biventricular hypertrophy are given in Box 4.

THE ABNORMALITIES OF THE Q WAVE

The Q wave normally is produced by septal activation from left to right. The characteristics of normal Q wave (< 0.04 in Q wave containing leads I, aVL and V_5–V_6) have already been discussed in normal electrocardiogram.

BOX 4: CRITERIA FOR BIVENTRICULAR HYPERTROPHY (Fig. 5.10)

- *Voltage criteria of LVH* (e.g. R wave > 27 mm in V_5 or V_6 and/or RV_5 + SV_1 > 35 mm associated with right axis deviation and clockwise rotation)

OR

- *Left ventricular hypertrophy* by voltage criteria as described above plus RVH in leads V_1 and V_2 ($R \geq S$ or $R : S \geq 1$) and a Katz-Wachtel phenomenon in mid-precordial leads (V_3–V_4)

- *Right ventricular hypertrophy* (RVH) by voltage criteria as discussed above plus left axis deviation.

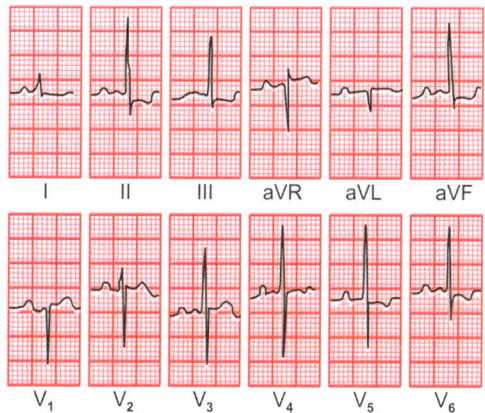

Fig. 5.10: Biventricular hypertrophy. There is right axis deviation (+75°). The R and S waves are of equal amplitude but larger than normal in leads V_3 and V_4 with voltage criteria of LVH (RV_5 + SV_1 > 35 mm). The good R wave in V_2 with large RS complex in V_3 indicates RHV. All these criteria suggest biventricular hypertrophy

What is an Abnormal Q Wave?

A Q wave greater than one small square in width (40 ms) and 2 mm in depth is considered as abnormal.

What is Significance of Q Wave?

As Q wave occurs due to septal activation, hence, septal infaction or septal hypertrophy will result in large Q wave.

Remember

Once an abnormal q wave is detected then look at ST segment and voltage of R wave in that leads.

- Presence of Q wave with ST elevation indicate acute myocardial infaction. If these changes are seen in anterior chest leads, then it is called *acute anterior wall infarction* and if present in inferior leads (leads II, III and aVF), then it is called *acute inferior wall infarction*.
- Presence of Q wave with large R wave in precordial leads (V_5–V_6) indicate left ventricular hypertrophy as seen in hypertrophic cardiomyopathy.

When does the Normal Q Wave Become Absent?

Normal Q wave becomes absent in left bundle branch block because now the septum is not activated from left to right.

What is Pathogenesis of Abnormal Q Wave?

Normally, the ventricle is depolarised from endocardium to epicardium, therefore, an electrode placed in the cavity of a ventricle would record only Q wave as a QS complex called negative complex of a cavity because all the depolarisation waves would be moving away from an electrode placed over it.

Now, think of a situation of myocardial infarction where a part of left ventricle is dead / necrosed and is electrically inert. This electrical inert portion creates an electrical window / hole through which an electrode placed at the surface peeps into the ventricle through this window and records Q wave of QS complex of a cavity. This pathogenesis has been discussed further in myocardial infarction.

What are other Common Causes of Q Wave?

A large number of conditions given in Box 5 produce noninfarction Q waves, hence presence of only Q wave without ST segment elevation and T wave inversion does not indicate infarction.

BOX 5: COMMON CAUSES OF NON-INFARCTION Q WAVE	
I. Myocardial diseases	*II. Pulmonary diseases*
• Myocarditis	• COPD
• Cardiac amyloidosis	• Pulmonary embolism
• Cardiac tumour	*III. Neuromuscular diseases*
• Hypertrophic cardiomyopathy	• Progressive muscular dystrophy
• Sarcoid heart disease	• Myotonia
• Dilated cardiomyopathy	• Friedreich's ataxia

THE ST SEGMENT ABNORMALITIES

Normally, the ST segment is isoelectric. It lies between the QRS complex and the T wave (Fig. 5.11A). It is assessed from the T-P line (an isoelectric line shown as dotted line in the Fig. 5.11A) for any deviation.

What are the Abnormalities of ST Segment?

Two abnormalities are:

1. The ST segment is too much elevated (more than normal) (Fig. 5.11B).
2. The ST segment is too much depressed (Fig. 5.11C).

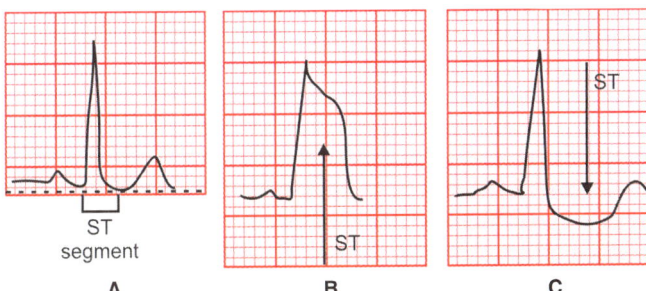

Figs 5.11A to C: Abnormalities of ST segment. (A) The ST segment is normally isoelectric; (B) ST segment elevation; (C) ST segment depression

What is Elevation of ST Segment? What is its Significance?

The isoelectric ST segment as already stated represents normally a state of repolarisation, hence, its deviation occurs due to repolarisation injury. The ST segment can be minimally elevated up to 2 mm in negroes. The elevation more than

BOX 6: CAUSES OF ST SEGMENT DEVIATION	
ST segment elevation	*ST segment depression*
• Acute myocardial infarction	• Acute subendocardial infarction
• Prinzmetal's angina	• Digitalis effect/toxicity
• Ventricular aneurysm	• Ventricular hypertrophy with strain
• Pericarditis and myocarditis	• Hypokalemia
• Early repolarisation syndrome (normal variant)	• Acute myocarditis
• Hyperkalaemia	• Mitral valve prolapse
• Hypothermia	• CVA
• Cardiac tumour	• Cardiomyopathies
• DC cardioversion	• Hyperventilation
• CVA	• Secondary ST-T change in bundle branch block, WPW syndrome and myocardial infarction (reciprocal change)

2 mm is abnormal and represents many conditions listed in Box 6. The ST segment elevation can occur normally in young persons; a condition called *early repolarisation syndrome*.

Pathogenesis of ST Elevation

The ST elevation expresses subepicardial injury / ischaemia or transmural ischaemia / injury, appears within minutes or hours of acute event. The ST segment is displaced upward from the baseline and its shape is coved or convexed. The 'J' point (at beginning of ST segment) is also elevated. This injury pattern represents the reduction of blood supply either due to coronary atherosclerosis or vasospasm (Prinzmetal's angina). In Prinzmetal's angina, the ST segment elevation occurs at rest during episode of pain and disappears with relief of pain.

Pathogenesis (Figs 5.12A and B): Since mean manifest ST segment vector is directed to the surface of injury (law of electrocardiography), the leads overlying the epicardial surface (e.g. lead V_5 shown) of injured myocardium reflects ST segment elevation (Figs 5.12A and B). The ST segment will be depressed in the lead V_1 as reciprocal change. The electrocardiographic effects of ischaemia / injury are represented in Figs 5.12A and B.

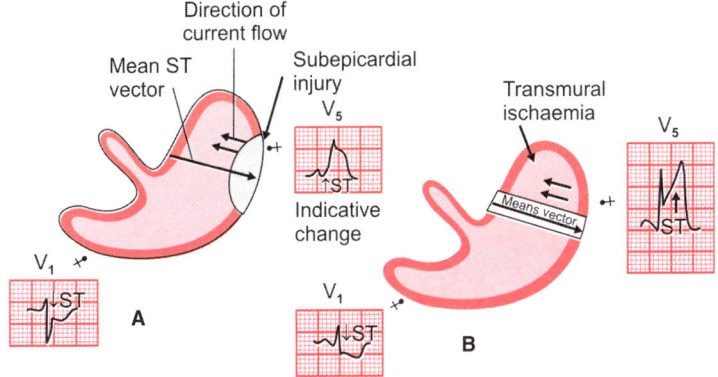

Figs 5.12A and B: The effect of (A) Subepicardial; (B) Transmural ischaemia/injury. ↑ST = Elevated ST segment. ↓ST means depression of ST segment

What does ST Segment Depression Mean?

The ST segment depression (Fig. 5.13) means the deviation of ST segment below the baseline, i.e. T-P line. Up to 0.5 mm ST segment depression can occur normally. Horizontal ST segment depression more than 0.5 mm staying for 80 ms (2 small squares) indicates myocardial ischaemia.

When ECG at rest is normal but symptoms suggest angina, a stress test is used to provoke ischaemia. The ST segment depression during stress test indicate effort induced angina. Positive stress test means ST segment depression > 1 mm during exercise.

Downslopping depressed segment as opposed to horizontal depression in the form of cup shaped depression called 'inverse tick mark sign' indicate digitalis effect or toxicity.

The causes of ST segment depression are given in Box 6.

GENESIS OF ST SEGMENT DEPRESSION

Myocardial Injury

When ischaemia becomes prolonged, it produces myocardial injury or damage. It is still reversible if blood flow to the area of ischaemia is restarted before death of tissue occurs; myocardial injury is reflected in ST segment change on ECG. The ST segment depression in subendocardial injury is in the form of 'J' point depression with either horizontally of ST

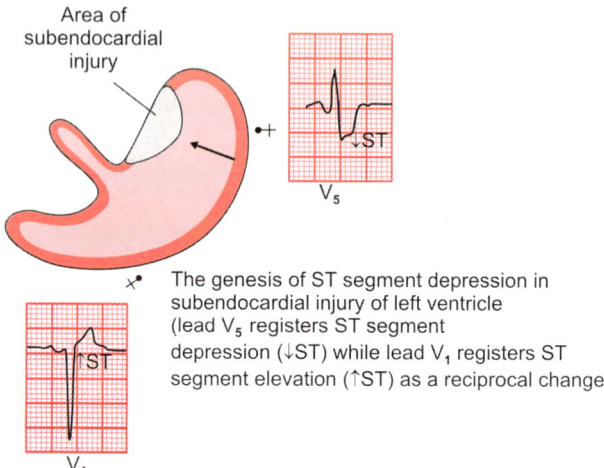

Area of subendocardial injury

The genesis of ST segment depression in subendocardial injury of left ventricle (lead V₅ registers ST segment depression (↓ST) while lead V₁ registers ST segment elevation (↑ST) as a reciprocal change

Fig. 5.13: The effect of subendocardial ischaemia on ST segment

segment or sagging ST segment or upward sloping or downsloping ST segment. The change is reversible if blood supply is restored in time. This is also called non-Q wave or subendocardial infarction (Fig. 5.13).

The ECG effects of myocardial injury

1. *The ST segment depression:* The ST segment depression is considered to reflect nontransmural or subendocardial ischaemia/injury. In the subendocardial ischaemic injury, the mean ST segment axis is directed towards the left ventricular cavity (Fig. 5.13) away from the epicardial surface (is away from leads V_5 and V_6), hence, ST segment depression is produced.

What is Angina? How does it Manifests on ECG

Angina is a pure clinical syndrome of chest pain of cardiac origin. It is due to transient disturbance due to reduced myocardial O_2 supply. It may or may not manifest on electrocardiogram. When it manifests, it produces ST segment depression in stable angina pectoris (Fig. 5.14). When angina is suspected but ECG is normal at rest, then stress ECG is advised to record ST segment depression on exercise (read stress electrocardiography).

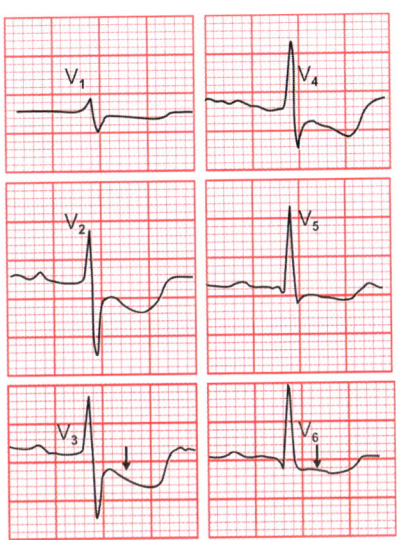

Fig. 5.14: Ischaemia of anterior wall. There is ST segment depression in precordial leads V_1–V_6 ($\downarrow$)

What is Prinzmetal's Angina?

It is a clinical syndrome of anginal pain accompanied by ST segment elevation during pain. The ECG change reverts back to normal with relief of pain.

What is ECG Change in Prinzmetal's Angina?

There is ST segment elevation instead of ST segment depression of stable angina (Figs 5.15A and B), hence called variant angina. Ischaemia of myocardium is due to vasospasm (vasospastic angina).

STRESS ELECTROCARDIOGRAPHY

What is Stress Electrocardiography? What is its Purpose?

Stress testing or electrocardiography is a noninvasive method to evaluate ischaemic heart disease, its severity and the effects of medical and surgical treatment and also used for rehabilitation of heart patients.

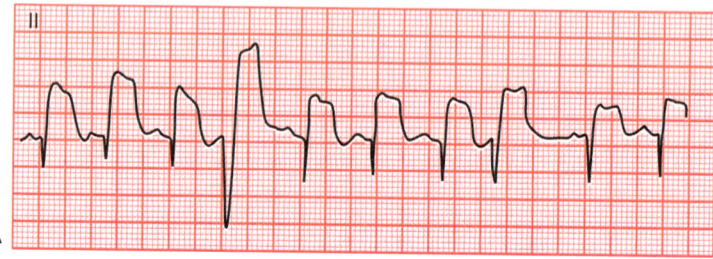

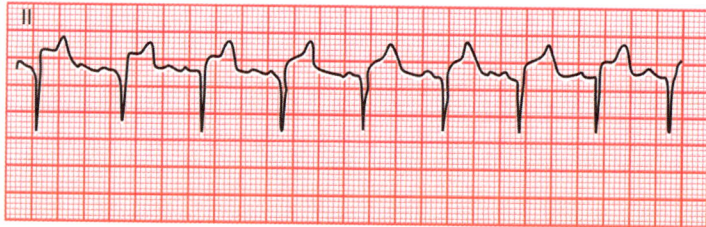

Figs 5.15A and B: Prinzmetal's angina. (A) The ECG lead II recorded during acute chest pain shows slope elevation of ST segment > 4 mm (inferior wall ischaemia due to vasospasm); (B) The same lead recorded immediately after relief of pain shows resolutions of ST change

The sole aim of exercise test is based on the principle that exercise increases myocardial oxygen demand, which although adequate at rest, becomes inadequate during exercise. Consequently, the ECG manifestations which were normal or equivocal at rest, become abnormal and significant during exercise indicating ischaemic heart disease.

Indications

1. To evaluate coronary artery disease in asymptomatic patients and in patients with atypical chest pain with normal ECG.
2. To evaluate the patients with postmyocardial angina.
3. For screening of asymptomatic patients who are at high-risk to develop IHD such as patients with diabetes, familial hyperlipidaemia, hypothyroidism, etc. It is also routinely employed for screening personnel after 40 yrs of age who are in special occupations (pilots, fire-fighters, police personnel, drivers and rail road engineers) and in those who

present themselves for a routine medical check up and applicants for life insurance.

4. To test effectiveness of treatment—a follow-up stress test is performed following coronary artery bypass surgery or coronary angioplasty.

5. *Left ventricular functional assessment:* During rehabilitation of acute MI, inducible ischaemia in this period indicates still viable and jeopardised myocardium. The decision to advise coronary angiography or revascularization depends on the results of these stress tests.

Stress testing is safe and noninvasive method to evaluate heart disease, to assess the functional progress and efficacy of treatment (medical or surgical).

Contraindications

1. Unstable angina with recent chest pain.
2. Uncontrolled cardiac arrhythmias.
3. CHF.
4. AV blocks.
5. Known severe coronary artery disease, e.g. left main coronary artery disease.
6. Impending or acute MI.
7. Critical aortic stenosis.
8. Uncontrolled hypertension.
9. Acute systemic illness.
10. Ventricular aneurysm.
11. Severe associated systemic disease such as pulmonary insufficiency, renal failure, uncontrolled diabetes, etc.

Methods

1. Bicycle ergometer
2. *Treadmill test* (Figs 5.16A and B): It is most commonly employed in Bruce protocol which employs initial higher workload with subsequent work increments at 3 minutes interval.

Lead system used is 12 lead surface ECG. Exercise test is terminated when patient develops symptoms and signs of myocardial ischaemia, i.e.

- Anginal pain or dyspnoea
- Drop in blood pressure or high BP response (systolic BP > 220 mm Hg)
- An arrhythmia.

What is Normal and Abnormal Stress Test?

Normal response to stress test on ECG include (i) increase in heart rate, (ii) shorter P-R and Q-T intervals, (iii) decrease in the height of R wave and (iv) minimal depression of upsloping ST segment (Figs 5.16A and B).

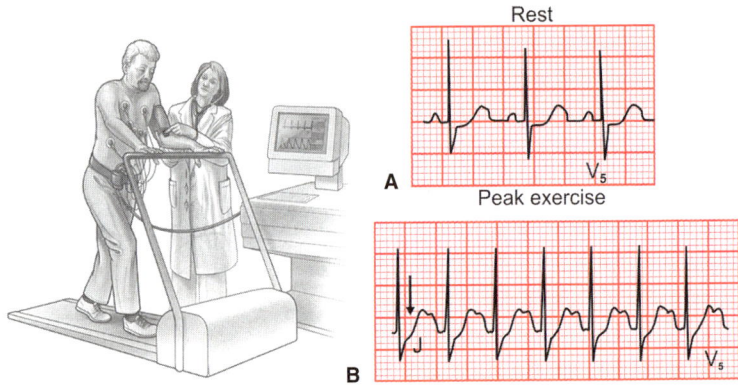

Figs 5:16A and B: Treadmill test, the ECG and blood pressure are continuously recorded as the patient walks in place on treadmill. The inclination of slope and speed of the treadmill are gradually increased during the test.

Normal ECG response to exercise: The lead V₅ recorded shows (A) At rest. The ST segment is isoelectric and normal; (B) At peak exercise. There is depression of 'J' point 2 mm during exercise (↓) with rapid upsloping ST segment. The upsloping ST segment is depressed by 1 mm for about 60 msec after 'J'point. This response is normal exercise response (read the text)

Treadmill test (Bruce protocol)					
Stage heart	Rest	02	1	2	3
Rate	90	125	136	152	170
BP	120/74	10/95	176/100	184/104	170/100

The abnormal response to stress include

- ST segment deviation (depression or elevation). The common change is ST depression > 1 mm staying for more than 0.08 sec or (0.80 ms; Fig. 5.17).
- Upsloping ST segment depression > 1.5 mm staying for > 0.08 sec (80 ms).

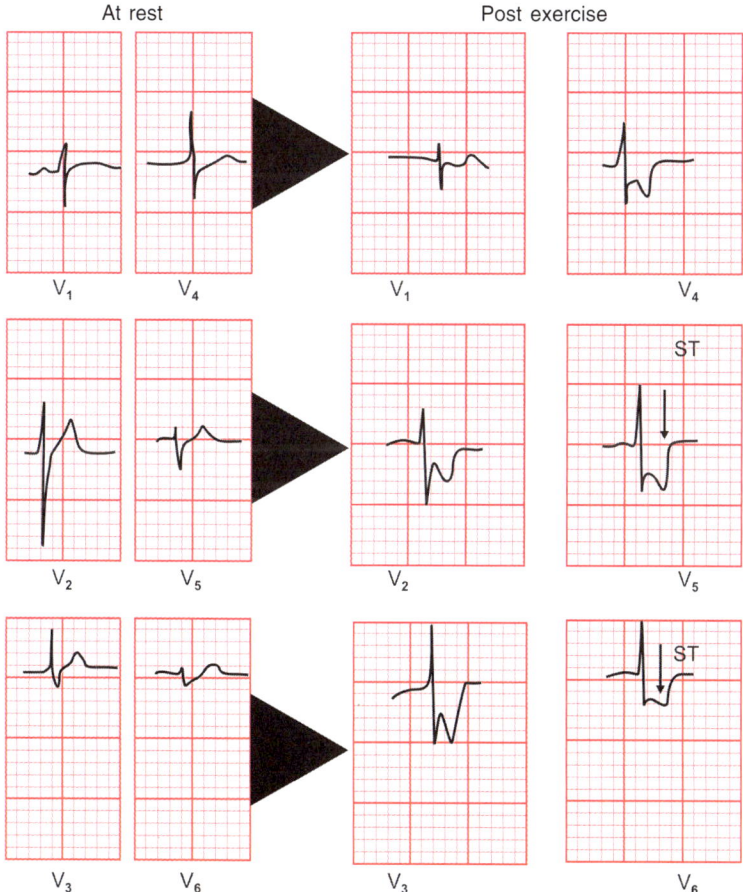

Fig. 5.17: Abnormal exercise response (positive stress test)

THE T WAVE ABNORMALITIES

The T wave represents the end of repolarization and it follows ST segment. The normal T is upright in leads where QRS complex is upright, i.e. leads I, II, III, aVL, aVF and V_3–V_6. It is normally inverted in leads aVR and V_1–V_2 and also in lead V_3 in some black persons.

Abnormalities of T Wave

- Too much tall
- Too much small or flat
- Inverted.

What is Tall T Wave? What are its Common Causes?

Normally, T wave is around 15% of the R wave in the same lead. T is said to be tall if it is more than one-third of the R wave. The causes of tall T wave are:

1. Early repolarisation syndrome (Fig. 5.18)
2. Posterior myocardial infarction
3. Hyperkalaemia
4. Scorpion bite
5. CVA (cerebrovascular accident)

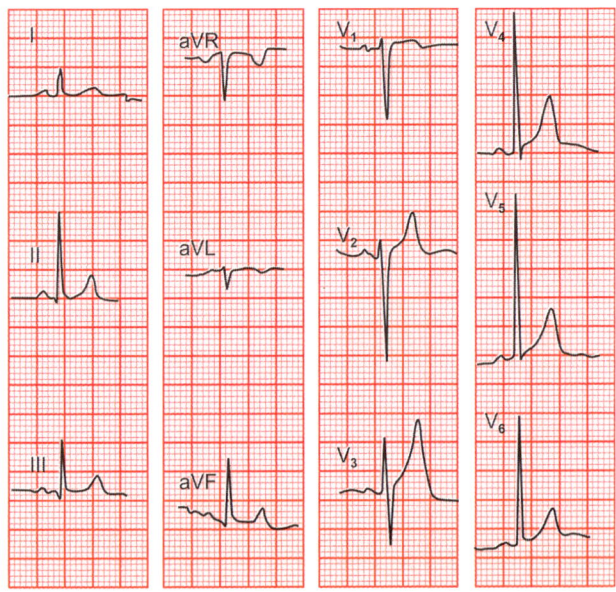

Fig. 5.18: Early repolarisation syndrome. Note the tall T waves in precordial leads

What is Small or Flat T Wave?

The T wave will be small or flat if QRS complex has low voltage (< 5 mm). The T wave may be small in electrolyte disturbance.

What is Inversion of T Wave?

Inversion of T means it is recorded below the baseline. The T wave inversion may be primary in cardiac disease where there is disturbance in repolarisation, e.g. myocardial ischaemia/infarction (Fig. 5.19) or secondary due to:

1. Subarachnoid hemorrhage (Fig. 5.20A)
2. Ventricular hypertrophy (Fig. 5.20B)
3. Bundle branch block
4. Myocarditis
5. Physiological conditions, e.g. heavy meal persistent juvenile pattern
6. Electrolyte disturbance
7. Digitalis toxicity (Fig. 5.20C)

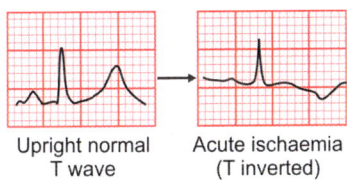

Upright normal   Acute ischaemia
T wave   (T inverted)

Fig. 5.19: Primary T wave change in acute ischaemia

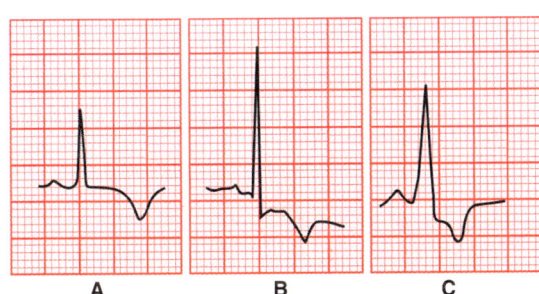

A   B   C

Figs 5.20A to C: Secondary T wave change. (A) Symmetric T wave inversion seen in cerebrovascular accident (subarachnoid haemorrhage); (B) Asymmetrical T wave inversion (the two limbs of T wave are unequal) seen in ventricular 'hypertrophy with strain; (C) The T wave inversion with ST depression (inverse tick mark sign) is seen in digitalis toxicity

MYOCARDIAL INFARCTION

Myocardial infarction is defined as the necrosis (death) of a part of the heart muscle due to critical reduction of blood supply due to sudden complete occlusion of a coronary vessel. Infarction involves virtually the left ventricle; right ventricular infarction is rare.

Classification

1. The Q wave infarction.
2. The non-Q wave infarction.

The presence of abnormal Q waves with other evolutionary changes (ST elevation and T wave inversion) is characteristic of acute myocardial infarction. The mere presence of Q wave does not signify infarction.

Pathogenesis of ECG Change in Infarcted Zone

The infarcted region of the myocardium consists of the three zones which are collectively called *ischaemia-injury-necrosis* zone (Fig. 5.21).

1. *Zone of necrosis:* This is the central area which is electrically negative, produces the Q waves/QS complex.
2. *Zone of injury:* The central zone of necrosis is surrounded by a zone of injury which produces ST segment elevation with convexity upwards.
3. *Zone of ischaemia:* This is outermost zone, produces ST depression with or without T wave inversion.

Since an electrode placed on the chest subtends a relatively large area, may include all the three zones and may reflect their ECG changes (Fig. 5.21), otherwise, all the three zones may be detected separately in different leads.

What is Myocardial Infarction Pattern on ECG?

1. A significant Q wave (QR or qR pattern) or QS complex in the leads recording infarction pattern.
2. The elevation of ST segment, hence called ST elevation myocardial infarction (STEMI).
3. Inversion of T wave.

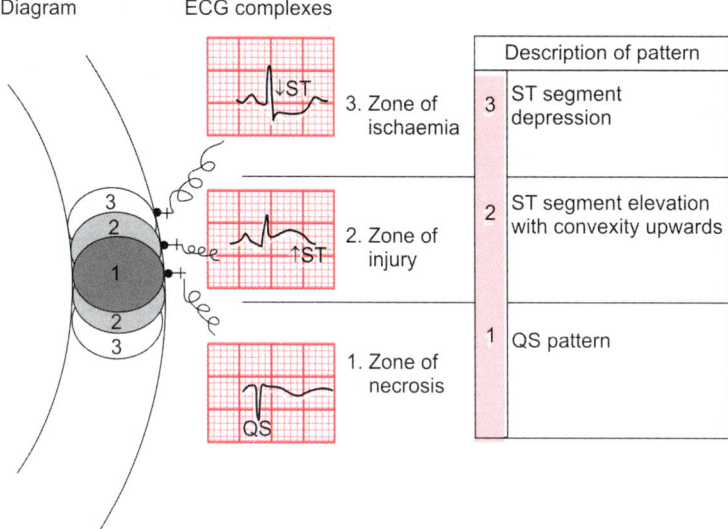

Fig. 5.21: The electrocardiographic manifestations of ischaemia-injury-necrosis sequence (diagram)

Remember

To say myocardial infarction is present, the above mentioned changes must be present in more than two adjoining (contiguous) leads.

Pathogenesis of Myocardial Infarction Pattern

Pathogenesis of QRS abnormalities

i. *A QS complex:* A QS complex is totally negative QRS, represents a complete loss of positivity and is recorded over the area of necrosis.

Pathogenesis: The myocardial necrotic tissue being electrically negative cannot be depolarised or activated, therefore, if it involves practically the full thickness of myocardium (transmural), a hypothetical electrical hole or a window is created in the ventricular wall. An electrode placed over this hole or window records negativity of surrounding muscle as well as that of cavity, thus records QS complex (Fig. 5.22C).

ii. *QR or qR complex:* A QR complex consists of a deep, wide abnormal Q wave followed a R wave; while in Qr, the abnormal Q is followed by a r wave, represents the depolarisation of viable myocardium in the infarcted ventricular free wall (Fig. 5.22B).

Pathogenesis: The significant loss of QRS forces will result in a pathological Q wave followed by late activation of viable myocardium that results in inscription of R(r) wave, the magnitude of which depends on the viable myocardium.

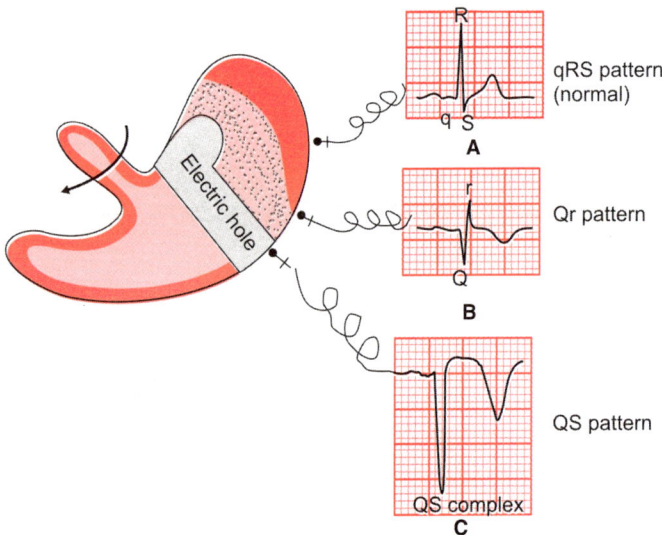

Figs 5.22A to C: Pathogenesis of (A) Normal qRS complex; (B) Diminished QRS activation following Q wave (Qr pattern); (C) The absent QRS activation (QS pattern)

The ST segment change

There is ST segment elevation with convexity upwards in the leads overlying the area of infarction (Figs 5.23A and B).

The ST segment elevation with coving/convexity upwards is the first ECG manifestation of myocardial infarction (epicardial injury). This ST elevation is seen in the leads overlying the infarcted area (Fig. 23A), hence, change is called *indicative change* (indicates the area infarcted). Conversely, a lead oriented towards the uninjured surface will record the

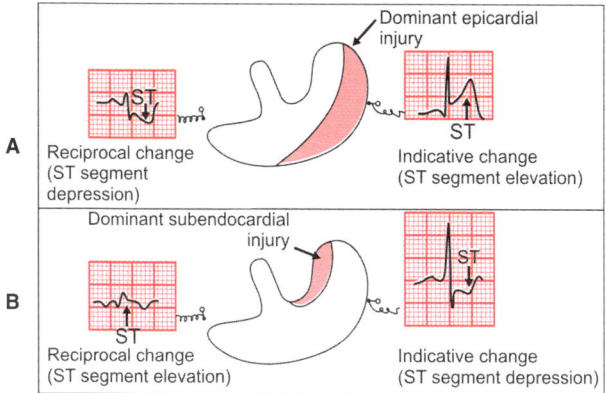

Figs 5.23A and B: Electrocardiographic changes. (A) Epicardial injury; (B) Subendocardial injury

opposite change (reciprocal of indicative change) i.e. depression of ST segment is called *reciprocal change* (Fig. 5.23A).

In subendocardial infarction, the ST segment depression is the indicative change and ST elevation becomes the reciprocal change (Fig. 5.23B). This is just reverse to transmural or subepicardial infarction.

The T wave change

Deep symmetric or asymmetric inversion of T wave accompanying ST segment elevation indicate myocardial infarction.

The inverted T wave may have isoelectric ST segment but shows an upward convexity called '*coronary T*' *wave* or may have slightly elevated ST segment above the baseline and upward convexity called *cove-plane T wave* (Fig. 5.24).

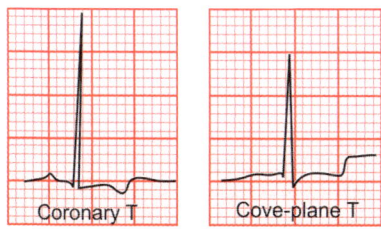

Fig. 5.24: T wave abnormalities in myocardial ischaemia/infarction

What is Evolution of Myocardial Infarction?

The first ECG abnormality seen in acute myocardial infarction (within few minutes to few hours) is ST elevation followed by appearance of Q wave and lastly there is inversion of T wave (Table 5.1 and Fig. 5.25). These changes may not evolve if patient is thrombolysed at the stage of ST elevation.

Q. What is hyperacute myocardial infarction? What is its significance?

Ans: Hyperacute myocardial infarction changes occur within few minutes to few hours (Fig. 5.26). These include ST segment elevation with dragged up T waves without evolution of Q waves. This is the stage where thrombolysis is indicated.

How do we Localise Myocardial Infarction?

The anatomical site of an infarction can be localised by the infarction patterns observed in specific leads (Box 7). A single lead is not diagnostic of an infarction. Left ventricular infarction is most common. Right ventricular infarct is rare.

Anterior Wall Infarction of Left Ventricle (Fig. 5.27)

Damage to the anterior wall of the left ventricle occurs usually due to occlusion of the left anterior descending artery. The ECG changes are usually reflected in precordial leads V_1 through V_6. Additionally there is loss of R wave height in these leads in association with abnormal Q wave, ST segment elevation and T wave inversion. Loss of R wave height in these leads is called *poor progression of the R waves*, may represent myocardial infarction.

The reciprocal ST segment depression in anterior wall infarction is seen in leads II, III and aVF.

In anteroseptal infarct: The ECG changes are seen in leads V_1–V_4 (Fig. 5.28).

Inferior Wall Infarction

Damage to the inferior (diaphragmatic) surface of the heart usually results from occlusion of the right coronary artery or less commonly the left circumflex coronary artery. The ECG

Table 5.1: The evolutionary changes of acute myocardial infarction

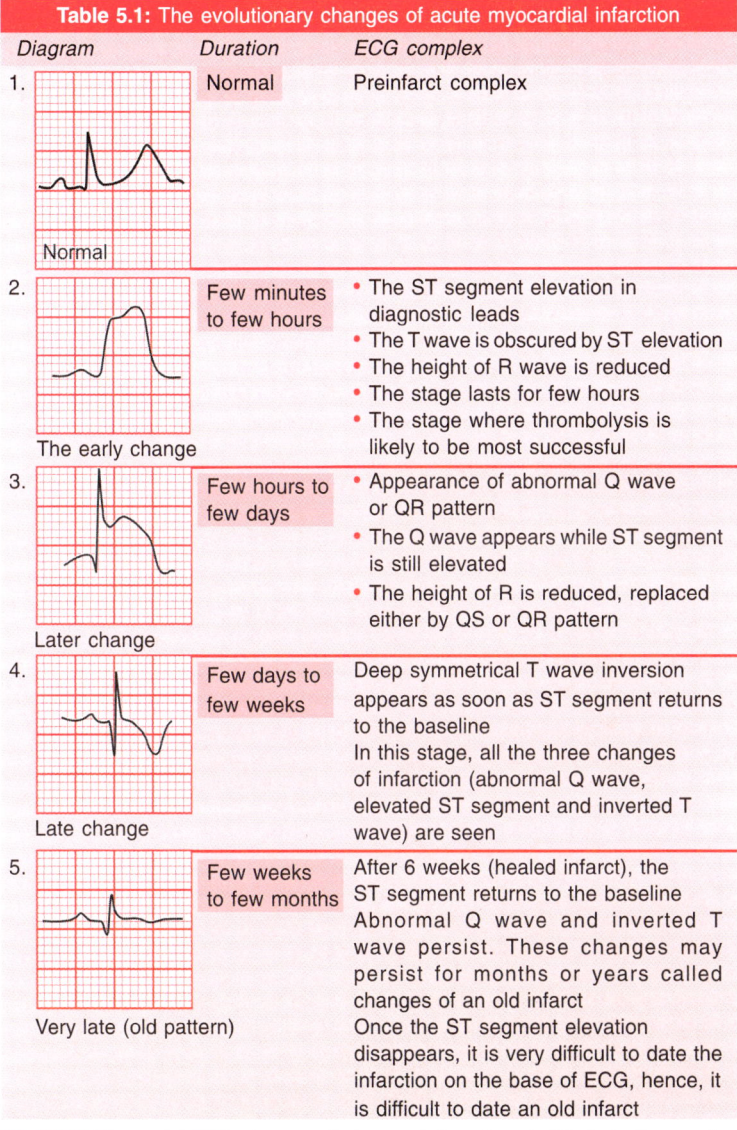

Diagram	Duration	ECG complex
1. Normal	Normal	Preinfarct complex
2. The early change	Few minutes to few hours	• The ST segment elevation in diagnostic leads • The T wave is obscured by ST elevation • The height of R wave is reduced • The stage lasts for few hours • The stage where thrombolysis is likely to be most successful
3. Later change	Few hours to few days	• Appearance of abnormal Q wave or QR pattern • The Q wave appears while ST segment is still elevated • The height of R is reduced, replaced either by QS or QR pattern
4. Late change	Few days to few weeks	Deep symmetrical T wave inversion appears as soon as ST segment returns to the baseline In this stage, all the three changes of infarction (abnormal Q wave, elevated ST segment and inverted T wave) are seen
5. Very late (old pattern)	Few weeks to few months	After 6 weeks (healed infarct), the ST segment returns to the baseline Abnormal Q wave and inverted T wave persist. These changes may persist for months or years called changes of an old infarct Once the ST segment elevation disappears, it is very difficult to date the infarction on the base of ECG, hence, it is difficult to date an old infarct

Fig. 5.25: The serial ECG changes during evolution of acute MI. A single complex is depicted. *Note:* The ECG changes do not appear simultaneously with infarction, take sometime to appear, therefore, ECG taken during acute chest pain due to infarction may be normal but a subsequent ECG taken after few hours may show changes. Hence, serial ECGs must be taken before a patient is declared not having an infarction

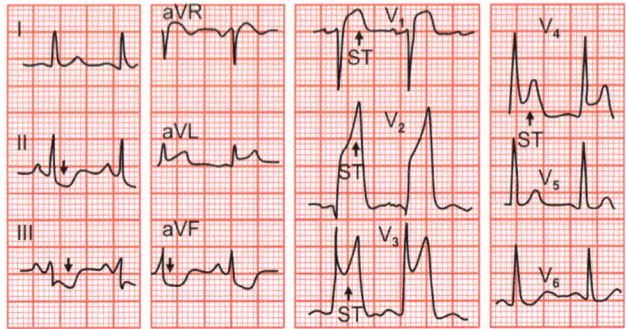

Fig. 5.26: Hyperacute anterior myocardial infarction (within 3 hrs.) There is acute ST elevation (↑ST) in leads V_1–V_4 with dragged up T waves without Q waves with reciprocal ST depression in leads II, III and aVF(↓). All these findings suggest hyperacute myocardial infarction where thrombolysis is likely to be successful

BOX 7: LOCALISATION OF MYOCARDIAL INFARCTION BY ECG	
Infarction of left ventricle	*Leads*
A. *Anterior wall*	(I, aVL and V_1–V_6)
• Anteroseptal	V_1–V_3 sometimes V_4
• Anterolateral	I, aVL and V_5–V_6
• Extensive anterior	I, aVL and V_1–V_6
B. *Inferior wall*	
• True inferior wall	II, III and aVF
• Inferolateral	II, III, aVF and V_5–V_6
C. *Posterior wall*	Mirror image change of infarction are seen in right precordial leads (V_{3R} and V_1)
• True posterior	V_{3R} and V_1–V_2
• Posterolateral	V_{3R}, V_1 and V_5–V_6

changes in inferior wall infarction are projected in leads II, III and aVF is called inferior surface oriented leads (Fig. 5.29).

At times, the reciprocal change (ST segment depression and T wave inversion) is seen in anterior leads I, aVL and V_1 to V_6 during acute MI.

☞ *The Q wave, ST segment elevation and T wave inversion is limited to leads II, III and aVF in inferior wall infarction. The reciprocal change may be present in leads I, aVL and V_1–V_6.*

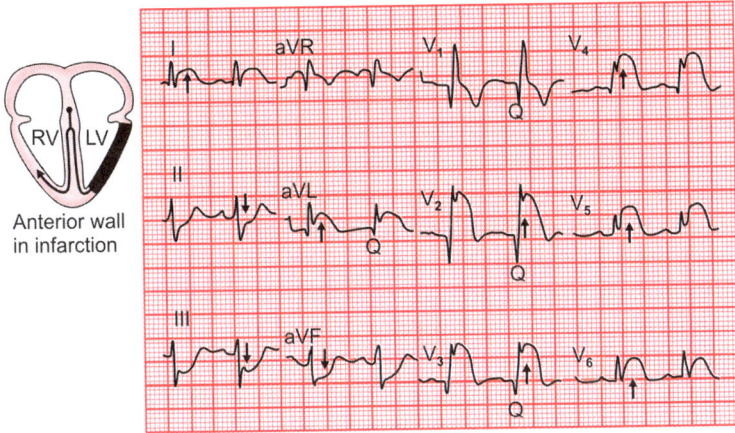

Fig. 5.27: Acute anterior myocardial infarction. The ECG shows (i) Marked elevation of ST segment with dragged up T waves in leads I, aVL and V_1–V_6 (↑); (ii) Reciprocal ST segment depressions in leads II, III and aVF (↓). There is q wave in leads aVL and V_1–V_4

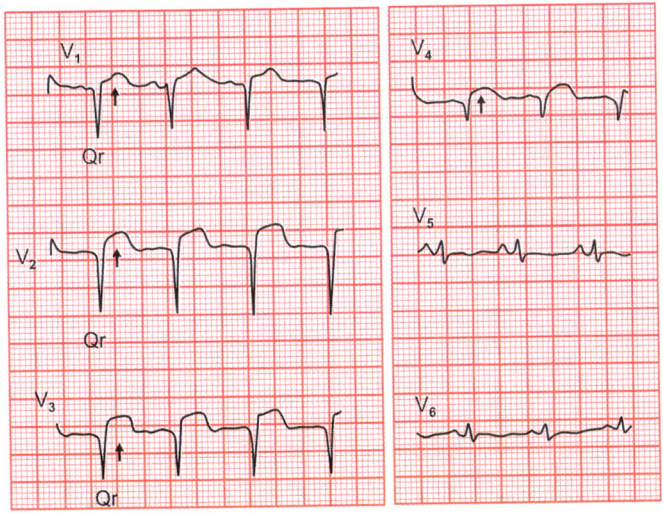

Fig. 5.28: Anteroseptal infarction. The ECG shows ST elevation in leads V_1–V_4 with dragged T waves. There is Qr pattern from leads V_1–V_4

If the infarction pattern extends from inferior wall to lateral wall, then it is called *inferolateral infarction*. It is reflected in leads II, III, aVF and V_5–V_6

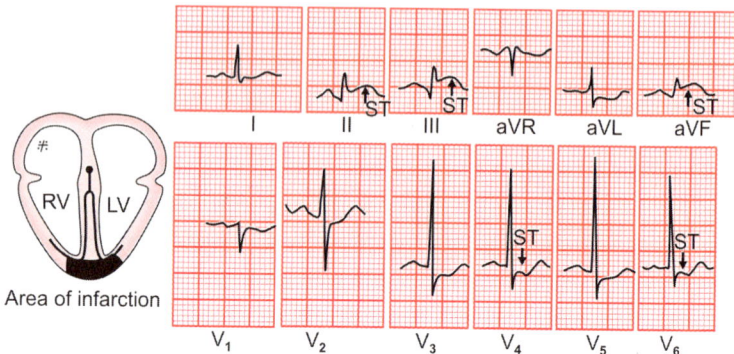

Fig. 5.29: Acute inferior wail Infarction. The ECG shows (i) The ST segment elevation (↑) is seen in leads II, III and aVF called inferior surface leads. This is indicative change of infarction; (ii) There is ST segment depression (↓) in anterior chest leads V_1–V_6 called reciprocal change

Posterior Wall Infarction

Remember that there is no conventional lead that represents the posterior wall of the infarction, hence, it is not the infarction pattern (abnormal Q wave, ST segment elevation and T wave posterior) which diagnose the inferior wall infarct, but the reverse of infarction change will be seen in the leads opposite to posterior wall, e.g. V_1 or V_2 (Figs 5.30A and B).

The ECG characteristics of posterior wall infarction will thus include (Fig. 5.31).

  i. The tall and wide R wave in V_1–V_2—this is mirror image change of QS complex seen in other infarctions.
 ii. The depressed concave upward ST segment. It is reverse of ST elevation seen in other infarction.
iii. The upright and tall T wave. This is reverse of deep symmetric T wave inversion.

An isolated true posterior wall infarction is unusual. Posterior wall infarction is almost accompanied either by inferior (e.g. leads II, III and aVF show infarction pattern in addition) or lateral wall infarction (leads V_5–V_6 show infarction pattern in addition) or both (e.g. ECG changes of posterior wall infarction are added to changes of inferior and lateral wall infarction).

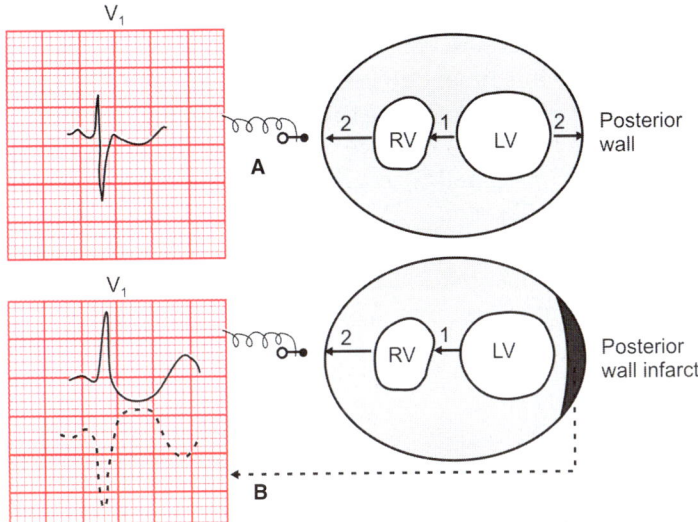

Figs 5.30A and B: Posterior wall infarction (diagrammatic illustration). (A) Normal ventricular depolarisation; (B) Ventricular depolarisation following posterior wall infarction producing tall, wide R wave with depressed concave upward ST segment and upright tall T wave (mirror image change of V_1 during infarction) shown below in the dotted lines. This change will only be picked up by the lead placed directly over the injured surface

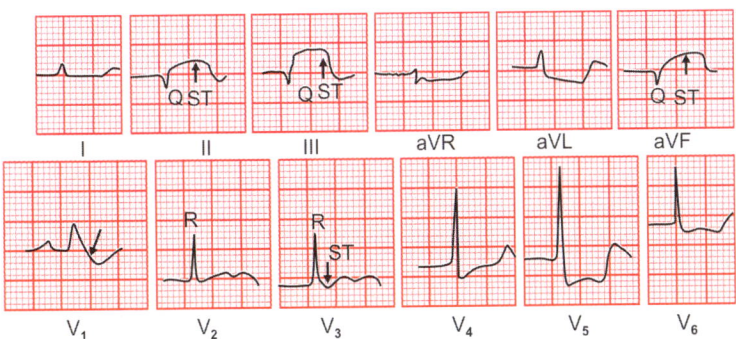

Fig. 5.31: Posterior wall infarction. The ECG shows (i) *Inferior wall infarction*. Note the ST segment elevation (↑) with q wave in leads II, III and aVF; (ii) *Posterior wall infarction*. There is a tall R wave with depressed ST (↓) segment and upright T wave (reciprocal of infarction pattern) in leads V_1–V_3; (iii) *Lateral wall ischaemia*. There is horizontal depression of ST segment from V_4 to V_6 indicating lateral wall ischaemia

What is an Old Infarct?

Since spontaneous healing of myocardial infarction takes 4–6 weeks, and by this time the ST segment has become isoelectric, therefore, an old infarct consists of the following changes:

i. Persistent abnormal Q wave.

ii. Isoelectric or normal ST segment.

iii. An inverted T wave.

These changes are seen in precordial leads in anterior wall infarction (Fig. 5.32) and in inferior leads (II, III and aVF) in inferior wall infarction (Fig. 5.33).

What is Subendocardial Infarction?

A subendocardial or also called non-Q wave infarction is characterized by persistent ST segment depression and T wave inversion. There is no Q wave. Infarction is established by raised biochemical markers of cardiac injury, e.g. CPK-MB and troponins.

The ECG characteristics (Fig. 5.34)

1. There is ST segment depression with deep symmetric T wave inversion.

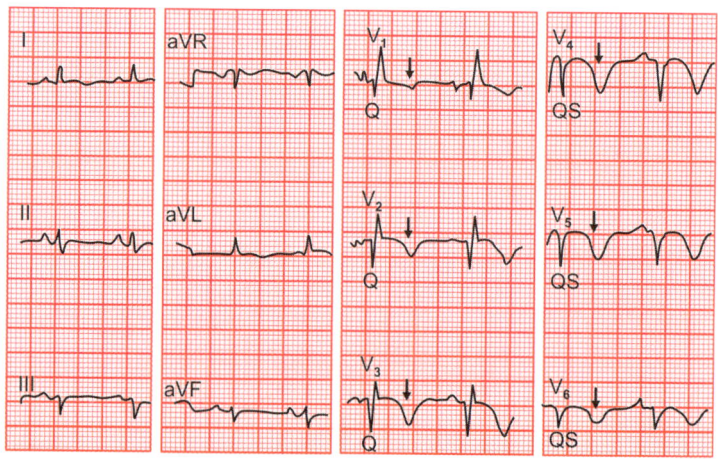

Fig. 5.32: Old anterior wall infarction. Note: ST segment is more or less isoelectric with deep symmetric T wave inversion (↓) in leads I, aVL and V_1–V_6. The height of R wave is reduced from V_1–V_6. Deep Q waves are present in leads V_1–V_3 while there is QS pattern in leads V_4–V_6

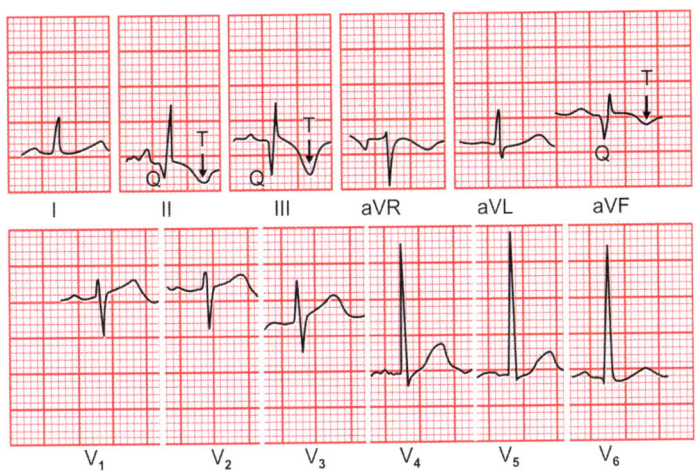

Fig. 5.33: Old inferior wall infarction. The ECG shows (i) The significant q waves with isoelectric ST segment and T wave inversion (↓) in leads II, III and aVF; (ii) The reciprocal change (ST depression) in anterior leads has disappeared

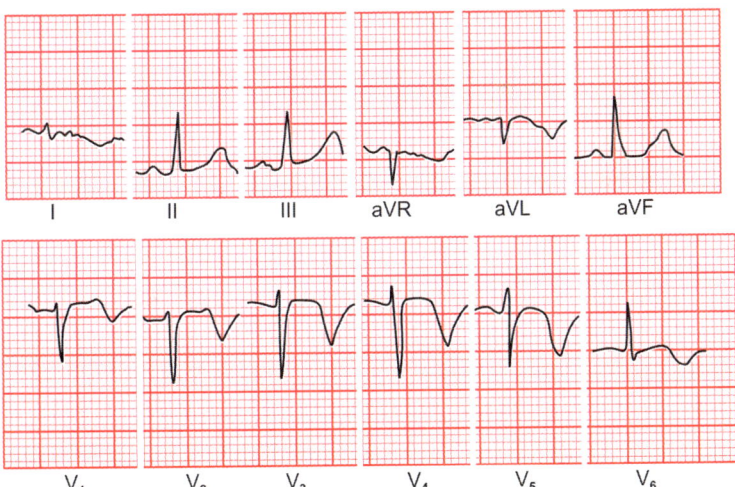

Fig. 5.34: Subendocardial infarction. The ECG shows deep symmetric T wave inversion, no Q wave and isoelectric ST segment in leads I, aVL, V₅ and V₆ indicating anterolateral subendocardial infarction

2. No change/alteration in morphology of QRS in these leads, i.e. there is no reduction in the height of R wave as seen in anterior wall infarction.

3. Absence of Q wave in these leads.

6
Electrocardiogram in Miscellaneous Conditions

- Myocarditis and pericarditis
- Pulmonary embolism (acute cor pulmonale)
- Chronic cor pulmonale
- Hypothyroidism
- Hypokalaemia and hyperkalemia
- Digitalis effect and toxicity
- Hypothermia

MYOCARDITIS

It is inflammation of the myocardium. It can be acute or chronic. Chronic myocarditis interchangeably used for dilated cardiomyopathy.

Infections (viral, bacterial, rickettsial, fungal, and parasitic) and some other conditions such as **radiation**, **drugs** and **chemical or physical injury** can result in myocarditis.

The ECG characteristics (Fig. 6.1)

- The ST segment elevation with concavity upwards (convexity of ST segment is observed in STEMI) and T wave inversion in precordial leads.
- The QT and QTc prolongation beyond 0.44 sec is characteristic.
- An arrhythmia or AV block (prolongation of P-R interval > 0.20 sec) is common.

Remember

Prolongation of QTc is gold standard for diagnosis of myocarditis.

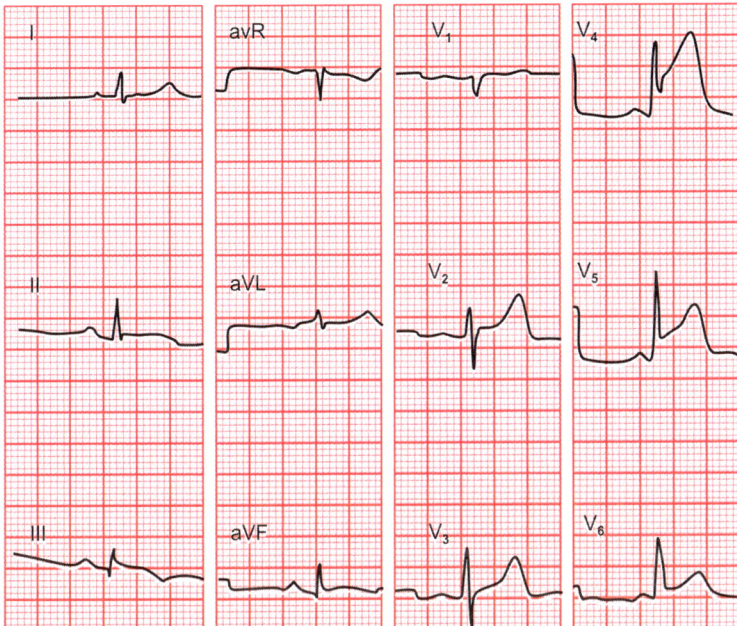

Fig. 6.1: Myocarditis. The ECG shows (i) Low voltage of QRS complexes in standard leads (I, II, III, aVR, aVL and aVF); (ii) There is slight prolongation of QT (QTc) interval; (iii) There is elevation of ST segment with concavity upwards in leads II, III, aVF and V_1–V_6. There is reciprocal ST depression in aVR

PERICARDITIS AND PERICARDIAL EFFUSION

Pericarditis is an inflammation of the pericardium, can be acute or chronic. A collection of fluid in the pericardium is called *pericardial effusion*.

Causes

The *causes* of pericarditis and pericardial effusion are:

1. *Infection,* e.g. viral, pyogenic and tubercular.
2. *Uraemic pericarditis* with or without effusion.
3. *Hypothyroidism (myxoedema):* It usually results in pericardial effusion.
4. *Neoplastic:* It is due to infiltration of pericardium by malignancy.
5. *Post-radiation*

6. *Trauma* or following cardiac surgery
7. *Collagen vascular disorders*
8. *Idiopathic*

The ECG characteristics (Fig. 6.2)

- The ST segment elevation with concavity upwards similar to myocarditis.
- The T wave is usually upright.

The ECG changes of myocarditis and pericarditis are more or less similar, hence, it is difficult to separate these two entities on ECG

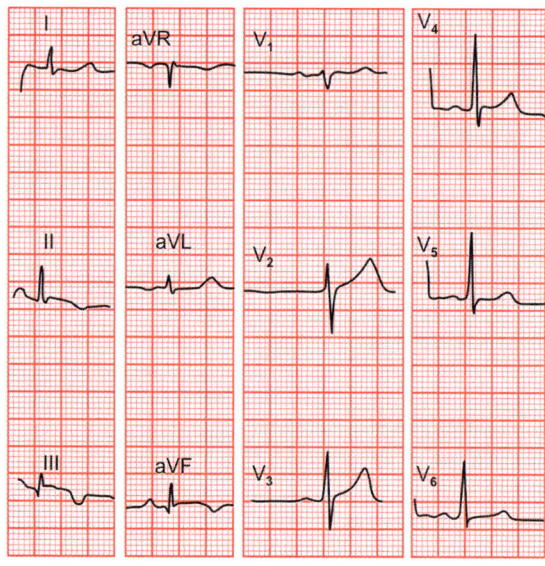

Fig. 6.2: Pericarditis. The ECG shows elevation of ST segment with concavity upwards in leads I, II, aVL, aVF and V_2–V_6 with ST depression in aVR

The ECG Characteristics of Pericardial Effusion (Figs 6.3A and B)

- *Low voltage graph:* The QRS complexes in the standard leads are < 5 mm in height and in chest leads < 10 mm in height.
- *Low to inverted T wave* in most of the leads.

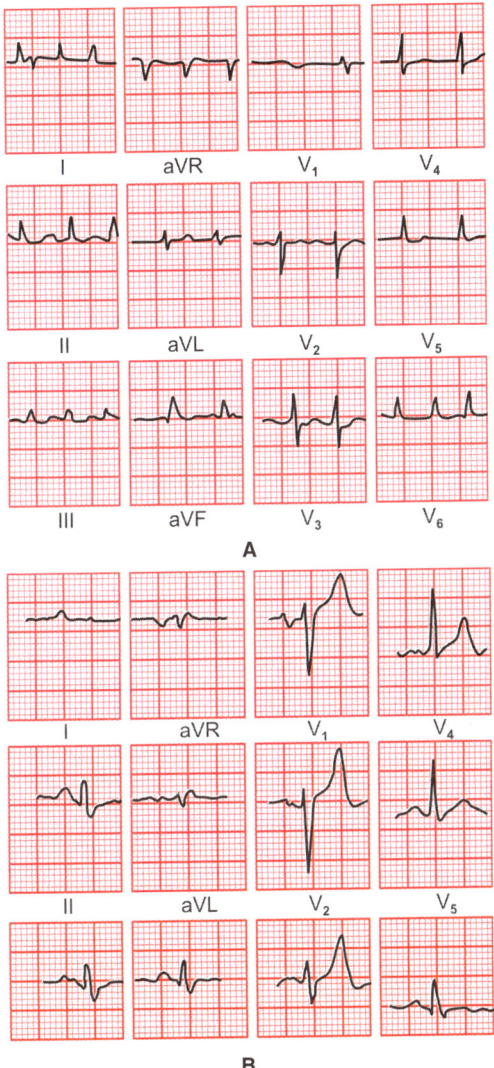

Figs 6.3A and B: Pericardial effusion:

(A) **Before paracentesis**

    (i) The low voltage graph (QRS < 5 mm in standard leads)

    (ii) Flat to law amplitude of T waves in most of the leads

(B) **After paracentensis**

    (i) Restoration of normal voltage

    (ii) Appearance of normal amplitude of T waves in precordial leads

- *Electrical alternans:* It is an electrical phenomenon in which the height of QRS alternates, i.e. one large QRS complex is followed by a small QRS complex. It is seen in massive pericardial effusion with cardiac tamponade. The QRS complex may also alternate in the polarity also, i.e. one upward complex is followed by a downward complex.

PULMONARY EMBOLISM

It is defined clinically as right ventricular hypertrophy or dilation secondary to development of acute pulmonary hypertension, often due to acute massive pulmonary embolism. It is characterized clinically by acute chest pain, haemoptysis and breathlessness in a patient with an evidence of peripheral vein thrombosis (cause of embolism).

The ECG characteristics

1. S_I Q_{III} and T_{III} syndrome (the classic triad of pulmonary embolism): This triad consisting of S wave in lead I and Q wave in lead III with an inverted T wave is seen less frequently than expected. These changes are transient, evolve within few hours of embolism and undergo resolution (Fig. 6.4).

2. *Acute right axis deviation of* > +110°. There may be clockwise rotation.

3. *Tall, peaked P waves (P-pulmonale)* are seen in standard leads, best in leads II, III and aVF due to right atrial hypertrophy.

4. *Transient RBBB pattern:* Incomplete (Fig. 6.4) or complete right bundle branch block (rSR' pattern in V_1 or V_2) may occur.

5. *Right ventricular hypertrophy with strain pattern* may be seen in leads V_1–V_2 (R:S ≥1 with ST depression).

6. *All types of atrial arrhythmias* (multiple atrial ectopics, multifocal atrial tachycardia, atrial flutter or fibrillation) can occur.

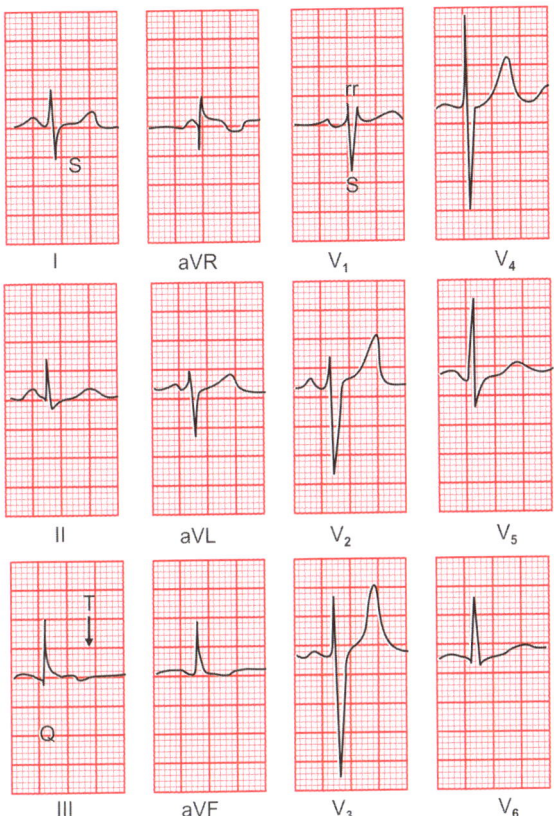

Fig. 6.4: Acute pulmonary embolism. The ECG recorded from a patient with acute thromboembolism shows (i) There was sinus tachycardia at a rate of 160 bpm (not shown); (ii) There is incomplete right bundle branch block (rSr' in V_1 a r wave in aVR and a wide S wave in V_5–V_6); (iii) There is an S wave in lead I, Q wave in lead III with an inverted T wave ($\downarrow$) constituting S_1, Q_{III} and T_m syndrome (labelled)

CHRONIC OBSTRUCTIVE PULMONARY DISEASE (COPD) AND CHRONIC COR PULMONALE

Chronic cor pulmonale clinically is defined as right ventricular hypertrophy or dilatation secondary to the disease of the lung parenchyma, pulmonary vasculature, thoracic cage and ventilatory control.

The ECG characteristics (Fig. 6.5)

1. Low voltage graph (QRS complexes are < 5 mm in standard leads) seen in predominant emphysema.
2. Right axis deviation (> + 90°) and clockwise rotation.
3. Right atrial hypertrophy (*P-pulmonale*)
4. Right ventricular hypertrophy
5. An arrhythmia, e.g. atrial ectopics and multifocal atrial tachycardia.
6. S_I, S_{II} and S_{III}, syndrome may sometimes be present.

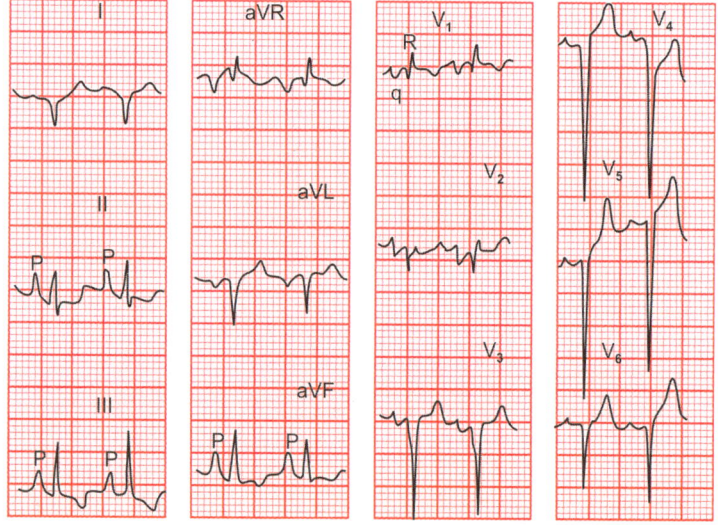

Fig. 6.5: Chronic obstructive pulmonary disease with chronic cor pulmonale. The 12 lead surface ECG shows (i) *Right axis deviation*; (ii) *Right atrial hypertrophy*. Note the tall P waves (>2.5 mm) in leads II, III and aVF (labelled). The P wave is biphasic in V_1–V_3 wherein the positive upward deflection is accentuated; (iii) *Right ventricular hypertrophy*. There is qR pattern in V_1 and V_2 with rS pattern from V_3–V_6 indicating nonprogression of R wave. This is due to marked clockwise rotation. In such a situation, the qRS of left ventricular complex will be recorded in leads V_7–V_9 if recorded (not shown here)

HYPOTHYROIDISM (MYXOEDEMA)

Cardiovascular findings in myxoedema include; slow pulse rate (bradycardia), cardiomegaly, conduction disturbances and pericardial effusion. These changes are due to hypometabolism and myxomatous infiltration into the heart and pericardium.

The ECG characteristics (Fig. 6.6)

1. *Slow heart rate or bradycardia* (HR < 60/min).
2. *Low voltage of QRS complexes* in standard leads (< 5 mm) is common. If there is an associated pericardial effusion, then there is generalised low voltage graph. The T wave also becomes flat.
3. *Conduction disturbance:* First degree heart block (P-R interval > 0.22 at HR of 60/min) is common. Other blocks are rare.
4. *Prolongation of QTc*
5. *The ST-T changes:* In hypothyroidism, the ST segment does not change and T wave may appear flat or low voltage. If there is significant ST segment depression and frank T wave inversion, then associated ischaemic heart disease may be suspected.

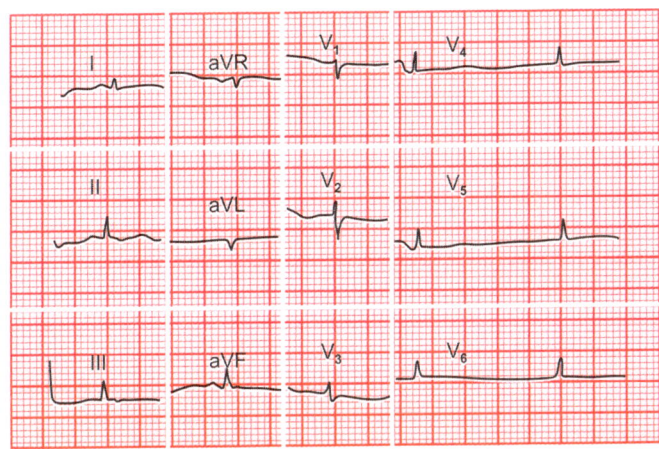

Fig. 6.6: Hypothyroidism. The ECG recorded from a patient of hypothyroidism shows (i) Generalised low voltage of QRS complexes; (ii) Slow heart rate (HR 62/min)

HYPOKALAEMIA (K⁺ < 3.5 mEq/L)

Potassium is the principal intracellular cation, takes part in depolarisation and repolarisation of cardiac cells membrane. Normal serum K^+ level is 3.5 to 5.5 mEq/L. Hypokalaemia is said to be present if K^+ is less than 3.5 mEq/L; while ECG changes usually appear when K^+ is < 3.0 mEq/L.

Causes

The causes are given in Table 6.1

Table 6.1: Causes of hypokalemia		
Gastrointestinal	**Renal**	**Miscellaneous**
• Low dietary intake	• Metabolic alkalosis	• Hypokalaemic
• Gastrointestinal loss:	• Diuretics	periodic paralysis
– Repeated vomiting	(loop diuretics)	• Insulin effect
– Diarrhoea	• Hyperaldosteronism	
– Fistulas	(primary) or	
– Ureterosigmoidostomy	secondary and Barter's	
	syndrome	
	• Liquorice ingestion	
	• Glucocorticoid excess	
	(iatrogenic, Cushing's	
	syndrome and ectopic	
	ACTH production)	
	• Renal tubular acidosis	
	• Renal tubular defects,	
	e.g. leukemia, Liddle's	
	syndrome and antibiotics	

The ECG characteristics (Fig. 6.7)

1. *Progressive diminution of the amplitude of T wave and increase in the amplitude of U wave.*

   The U wave that represents delayed repolarisation, occurs after the T wave and becomes prominent as hypokalaemia increases in severity; and on the other hand, the height of the R wave diminishes. The prominent U wave comes near to the T wave and even may become equal or larger than T wave. Sometimes, it may fuse with the T wave to form 'TU' complex (Fig. 6.7) from where it is difficult to separate T from U wave. The prominence of U wave is not sine qua non of hypokalemia but is suggestive of it.

   Low amplitude of T wave and prominent U wave or fusion of T and U wave (TU complex) is seen in hypokalaemia.

2. *Prolonged QTU interval while Q-T interval remains normal* (Fig. 6.7): In hypokalaemia, the U wave becomes prominent and gets superimposed on T wave in such a way that it gives

false impression of wide T wave instead of TU complex, giving a misinterpretation of prolonged QT; while in fact in other leads, where T and U are clearly defined and Q-T interval remains normal.

3. *The ST segment depression* in all the leads.
4. *Prolongation of P-R interval* or first degree AV block.
5. *Arrhythmias* (atrial premature complexes, ventricular premature complexes, VT and ventricular fibrillation).

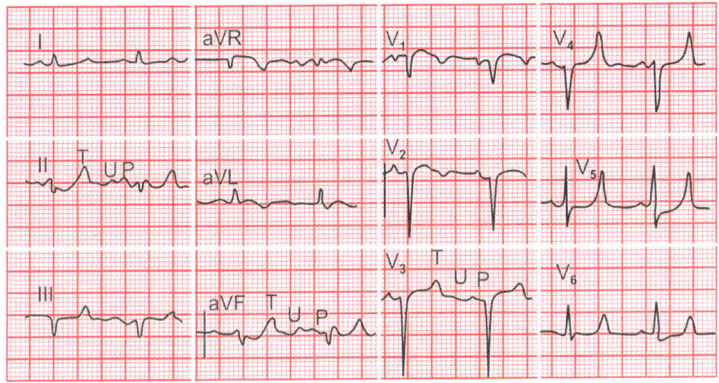

Fig. 6:7: Hypokalaemia (serum K⁺ 2.2 mEq/L). The ECG shows (i) There is diminished amplitude of T wave with prominent U wave best seen in precordial leads; (ii) Prolongation of QTU or QTc interval; (iii) Fusion of T and U wave as TU complex seen in leads II and aVF; (iv) 'TUP' complex. Due to prolongation of QTU interval, the P wave comes, near to TU waves forming TUP complex seen in leads II, aVF and V_3 (labelled)

HYPERKALAEMIA (SERUM K⁺ > 5.5 mEq/L)

An increase in level of serum K⁺ above 5.5 mEq/L is termed as *hyperkalaemia*. The ECG changes appear when the serum level of K⁺ arises above 6.0 mEq/L. It is not necessary to have ECG changes in all patients of hyperkalaemia.

Causes

The causes are summarised in Table 6.2.

The ECG characteristics (Fig. 6.8)

There is good correlation between rise in serum K⁺ levels and ECG changes. The ECG, actually reflects the gradients between myocardial intracellular and extracellular potassium ions. The

Table 6.2: Causes of hyperkalaemia

1. *Inadequate excretion*
    a. Renal failure (uraemia)
    b. Adrenal insufficiency, e.g. hypoaldosteronism and Addison's disease
    c. Potassium-sparing diuretics, e.g. spironolactone and triamterene
2. *Shift of potassium from tissues into circulation*
    • Crushed muscle injury (rhabdomyolysis)
    • Haemolysis
    • Internal bleeding
3. *Drugs*, e.g. succinylcholine and beta blockers
4. *Acidosis*
5. *Hyperosmolality*
6. *Diabetic ketoacidosis*
7. *Hyperkalaemic periodic paralysis* (inherited)
8. *Excessive K^+ intake* (K^+ salts or juice)

abnormality involves the P wave, the QRS, the T wave and the ST segment.

1. *Tall, peaked T waves* present in precordial leads (Fig. 6.8) are best seen in leads V_2–V_3. Hyperkalaemia shortens repolarisation, i.e. T wave comes near to QRS.

   Peaking of T wave is the earliest sign of hyperkalaemia.

2. *The widening of QRS:* The amplitude of R wave decreases and total duration of QRS increases with rise in K^+ levels.

   The QRS becomes wider and wider with rise in K^+ levels.

3. *The QRS-T fusion (a sine-wave pattern):* When the K^+ level is markedly high, the progressive widening of QRS and T wave brings the T wave near to QRS complex or even fusion may occur.
4. *Shortening of QTc* interval (< 0.36).
5. *ST-T wave change:* There is ST segment depression but the T wave remains upright.
6. *Wide and flat P waves:* With progressive rise in K^+, the amplitude, of P wave decreases and its width increases. At times, P wave is not visible (atrial standstill).

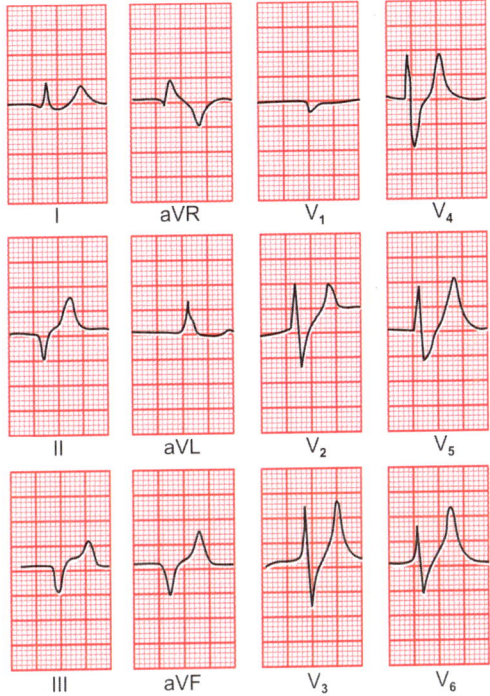

Fig. 6.8: Hyperkalaemia (serum K^+ was 6.2 mEq/L). The ECG shows (i) Tall tented T waves in all leads especially the precordial leads; (ii) There is associated ST depression with tall T wave; (iii) The QTc is shortened; (iv) The P wave are of low amplitude or invisible in leads I, aVL and V_1–V_6

7. *P-R interval:* It is usually normal, but gets prolonged with marked rise in serum K^+.

8. *Ventricular arrhythmias* (e.g. VT, ventricular flutter and asystole).

DIGITALIS

It is a cardiac glycoside used in the treatment of congestive heart failure and supraventricular tachycardia.

Actions

1. Positive inotropic effect.
2. Negative chronotropic effect.
3. Augments automaticity (enhance excitability).
4. Prolongation of effective refractory period of the heart.

The ECG characteristics

Digitalis is used to enhance myocardial performance in chronic congestive heart failure as well as to control many supra-ventricular arrhythmias. Normal serum levels (1–1.5 ng/L) of digoxin produce certain effects on ECG called *digitalis effect*; while higher levels (> 2 to 3.0 ng/L) produce life-threatening arrhythmias, heart blocks and other significant side-effects called *digitalis toxicity*. The ECG in digitalis effect and in digitalis toxicity is discussed separately because in digitalis toxicity, the ECG changes of digitalis effect are present in addition to digitalis induced arrhythmias or heart blocks.

The digitalis effect (Figs 6.9 and 6.10)

1. *Inverse check mark configuration of ST segment* (Fig. 6.9): The ST segment is scooped out and assumes the shape of inverse check mark sign (mirror image of check mark) a characteristic feature of digitalis effect.
2. *Elevated ST segments* in leads where the main QRS deflections is negative (e.g. lead V_1).
3. *Flattening or inversion of T wave:* The digitalis diminishes the amplitude of T wave with the result it may become flattened. The inversion of T wave occurs in digitalis toxicity.
4. *Shortening of QTc interval.*
5. *Prolongation of P-R interval* as compared to pretreatment baseline. The P-R interval lengthens but does not go beyond

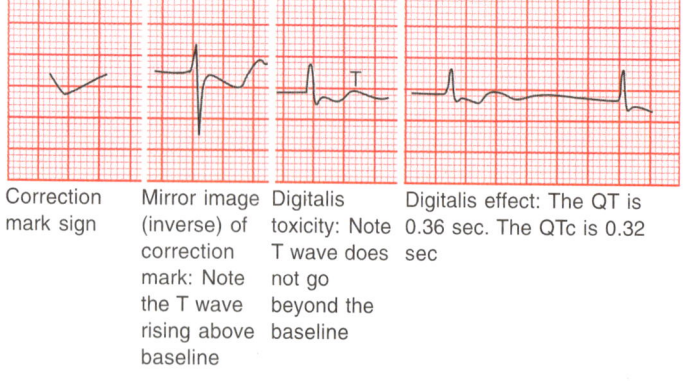

| Correction mark sign | Mirror image (inverse) of correction mark: Note the T wave rising above baseline | Digitalis toxicity: Note T wave does not go beyond the baseline | Digitalis effect: The QT is 0.36 sec. The QTc is 0.32 sec |

Fig. 6.9: Digitalis effect and digitalis toxicity (diagram)

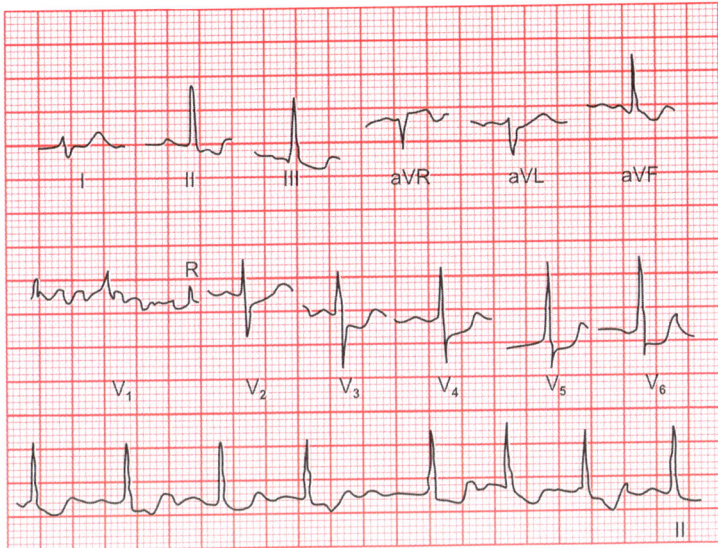

Fig. 6.10: Digitalis effect. The 12 lead surface ECG recorded from a patient with rheumatic heart disease with mitral stenosis taking digitalis shows (i) *Right axis deviation*; (ii) *Right ventricular hypertrophy*. There is tall R wave in V_1 and V_2 (R:S > I) with persistence of S wave in V_5–V_6; (iii) *Atrial fibrillation*. Note the undulation of baseline due to fibrillatory (f) waves in lead V_1. The lower strip of lead II shows fibrillatory (f) waves, undulation of the baseline and variable R-R intervals; (iv) *Patient was receiving digitalis for atrial fibrillation*. Note the characteristic ST segment depression in the form of inverse check mark sign, seen in all the leads—a characteristic of digitalis effect

0.22 sec at heart rate of 60/min. First degree heart block (P-R > 0.24 sec) is called *digitalis toxicity* rather than digitalis effect.

6. *Fall in heart rate:* Digitalis slows the heart rate and even bradycardia may occur.

The Digitalis Toxicity

It is common with digitalis use because of narrow margin of safety. The hypokalaemia, old age, hypoxaemia, magnesium depletion, renal and hepatic insufficiency, hypothyroidism, hypercalcaemia and electrical cardioversion are the common precipitating factors. Chronic digitalis intoxication is insidious onset, is characterised by:

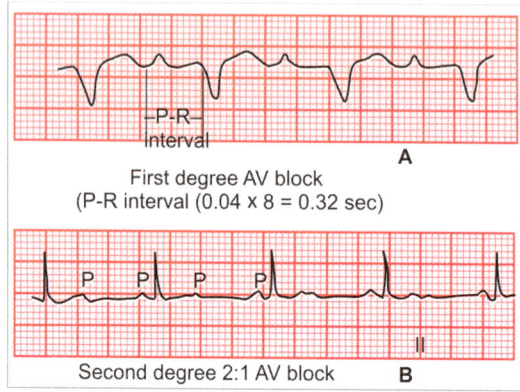

First degree AV block
(P-R interval (0.04 x 8 = 0.32 sec)

Second degree 2:1 AV block   **B**

Figs 6.11A and B: Conduction disturbances due to digitalis toxicity

1. *Extracardiac manifestations,* e.g. weight loss, cachexia, nausea, vomiting, neuralgia, gynaecomastia, yellow vision and delirium.
2. *Cardiac manifestations* include exacerbation of heart failure, arrhythmias (digitalis induced arrhythmias), heart blocks, etc.

The ECG characteristics (Figs 6.11 and 6.12)

1. All the ECG characteristics of digitalis effect are present, e.g. inverse check mark shape of ST segment, shortening of QTc and prolongation of P-R interval.
2. The T wave inversion with inverse check mark shape of ST segment indicates digitalis toxicity not the effect.
3. *AV blocks* (Figs 6.11A and B): The first degree AV block is common. Supraventricular tachycardia (nonparoxysmal) with block is the characteristic feature of digitalis toxicity. All grades of blocks are known to occur in digitalis toxicity.
4. *Arrhythmias* (Fig. 6.12). These include:
   - *Atrial,* e.g. atrial ectopics, paroxysmal atrial tachycardia with AV block and atrial bigeminy.
   - *AV nodal,* e.g. ectopics, junctional escape rhythm and accelerated AV nodal rhythm.
   - Ventricular, e.g. ventricular ectopics, ventricular couplets, ventricular bigeminy, ventricular tachycardia etc.

HYPOTHERMIA

Hypothermia (low core body temperature) may be a complication of cold exposure and is aggravated by taking

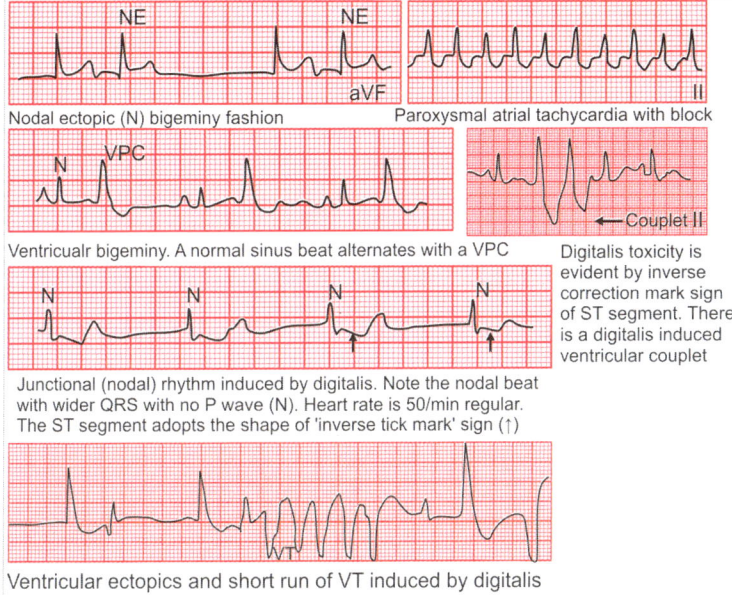

NE NE

aVF II

Nodal ectopic (N) bigeminy fashion

Paroxysmal atrial tachycardia with block

N VPC

←Couplet II

Ventricualr bigeminy. A normal sinus beat alternates with a VPC

Digitalis toxicity is evident by inverse correction mark sign of ST segment. There is a digitalis induced ventricular couplet

N N N N

Junctional (nodal) rhythm induced by digitalis. Note the nodal beat with wider QRS with no P wave (N). Heart rate is 50/min regular. The ST segment adopts the shape of 'inverse tick mark' sign (↑)

Ventricular ectopics and short run of VT induced by digitalis

Fig. 6.12: Digitalis induced arrhythmias

vasodilator drugs and drinking alcohol. The causes are given in Box 1. Hypothermia may be induced in conjunction with cardiac surgery or other procedure.

The ECG characteristics (Fig. 6.13)

Prolonged exposure to critically low temperatures (< 35°C) will profoundly depress both the electrical and mechanical activity in the heart. The ECG changes in hypothermia are variable and include:

1. Sinus bradycardia (core temp. 35° to 37°C).
2. Prolonged P-R interval (core temp. 30° to 35°C).
3. Widening of QRS interval (core temp. 30° to 35°C).
4. Lengthening of ST segment and Q-T interval (core temp. 30° to 35°C).
5. *Osborn wave (also called osborn J waves):* This wave is seen as a notch or depression in the terminal portion of QRS (descending limb of R wave) when core temperature falls below 30°C.

Osborn wave is characteristics of hypothermia when core body temperature is < 30°C.

6. Ventricular arrhythmia (core body temp. less than 30°C).

BOX 1: CAUSES OF HYPOTHERMIA

A. Accidental hypothermia (due to cold exposure in winter months)

- Myxoedema
- Pituitary insufficiency
- Addison's disease
- Hypoglycaemia
- CVA
- Wernicke's encephalopathy
- Myocardial infarction
- Ingestion of alcohol or pancreatitis
- Cirrhosis of the liver

B. Hypothermia secondary to acute illness

- CHF
- Uraemia
- Drug overdosage
- Diabetes mellitus

C. Immersion hypothermia

Deep cold water swimmers

D. Induced hypothermia

- Cardiac surgery
- Other procedures

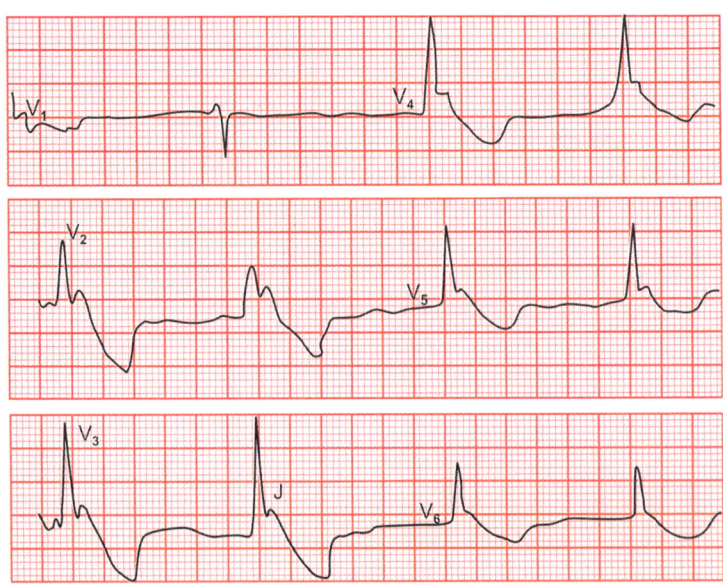

Fig. 6.13: Hypothermia. Osborn J wave are seen. There is lengthening of ST segment and Q-T interval

7

Self-Assessment (Test yourself)

- How to report an ECG?
- Normal ECG at glance
- Self-interpretation of ECGs

Since you have learnt every aspect of ECG, now test yourself. You should now be able to recognise the common ECG patterns. Two important things should be remembered while interpreting an ECG.

1. The ECG belongs to an individual patient, hence, must be interpreted in the light of patient complaints.
2. Interpretation of ECG must be correlated with the clinical picture of the patient before contemplating intervention.

HOW TO REPORT AN ECG?

ECG should be reported in a systematic manner as reported in the proforma (Box 1).

BOX 1: PROFORMA FOR ECG		
Name	*Age and sex*	*Clinical Diagnosis*
• Rhythm and Heart rate		
• Cardiac axis		
• P wave and P-R interval		
• QRS complexes (e.g. Height, widths Q wave duration)		
• ST segment		
• T waves		
• ECG diagnosis		

NORMAL ECG AT GLANCE

The Normal Durations

1. P-R interval < 0.20 sec (five small squares)
2. QRS duration < 0.12 sec (120 ms or 3 small squares)
3. QTc interval < 0.44 sec.

Normal Axis

0° to 90°

P Wave

Normal P wave is < 2.5 mm in height as well as in duration.

Height of R Wave in QRS Complex

- R wave in V_1 is less than S wave
- R wave in V_5 is < 25 mm
- $RV_5 + SV_1 < 35$ mm

ST Segment

Isoelectric

T Wave

- Less than 15% of R wave
- Tall T means 75% of R wave
- T is upright in all the leads except aVR, V_1 and V_2.

HOW TO READ AN 12-LEAD ECG?

Hold the ECG between your two hands and start reading from the left side:

1. First of all look at the standardisation inscribed in the beginning of ECG. Normal standardisation is 10 mV (10 small squares). Half standardisation is 5 small squares and double standardisation means 20 small squares.
2. *Look at the rhythm, i.e. R-R interval:* Is rhythm regular or irregular? Calculate the heart rate (1500 ÷ R–R if HR is regular).
3. *Look at the axis:* Note, whether axis is normal or abnormal (right or left) by looking at standard leads.
4. *Look at the electrical rotation:* For this look at the precordial leads (V_1–V_6). Find out the transition zone (R = S in transition

zone). Note, whether this zone lies normally (V_3 or V_4) or displaced to the right (counterclockwise rotation) or left (clockwise rotation).

5. *Look at the P Wave*
   - Normal P wave is < 2.5 mm in height and width.
   - Tall P wave > 2.5 mm indicates right atrial hypertrophy.
   - Wide P wave > 2.5 mm indicates left atrial hypertrophy.

6. *Now look at QRS complex*
   - Find whether there is an Q wave, if present, note the lead. Is Q wave normal or abnormal? Normally a q wave is present in Q wave containing leads, i.e. leads I, aVL and V_5–V_6.
   - Calculate the width of QRS (normal is 0.05 – 0.09 sec), wide QRS (> 0.12 sec) indicates bundle branch block.
   - Find the voltage/height of R wave. Normally, R wave is less than S in V_1 and < 25 mm in V_5. Tall R wave in V_1 indicates right ventricular hypertrophy while tall R wave in V_5 (> 27 mm)indicates left ventricular hypertrophy.

Look at P-R interval

- Is it normal or prolonged or short. (Normal P-R is 0.12–20 sec). P-R interval > 0.20 sec indicates first degree AV block, while short P-R interval < 0.10 sec indicates WPW syndrome.
- Now look whether there is one P for each QRS or there are more P than QRS.

  Normally, there is one P for each QRS. More P than QRS indicate heart blocks.

Now look at ST segment

- Isoelectric ST segment is normal.
- Elevated ST indicates myocardial infarction or Prinzmetal's angina.
- Depressed ST indicates ischaemia, digoxin toxicity and electrolyte abnormality.

Now look at T wave

- Tall peaked T waves are seen in hyperkalemia, posterior wall infarction and early repolarisation syndrome.
- Inverted T indicates ischaemia infarction or ventricular hypertrophy or BBB.

SELF INTERPRETATION OF ECG

ECG 1

A young man presented with palpitation and dyspnoea. He landed in the emergency and casualty department in congestive heart failure where the ECG was recorded (displayed).

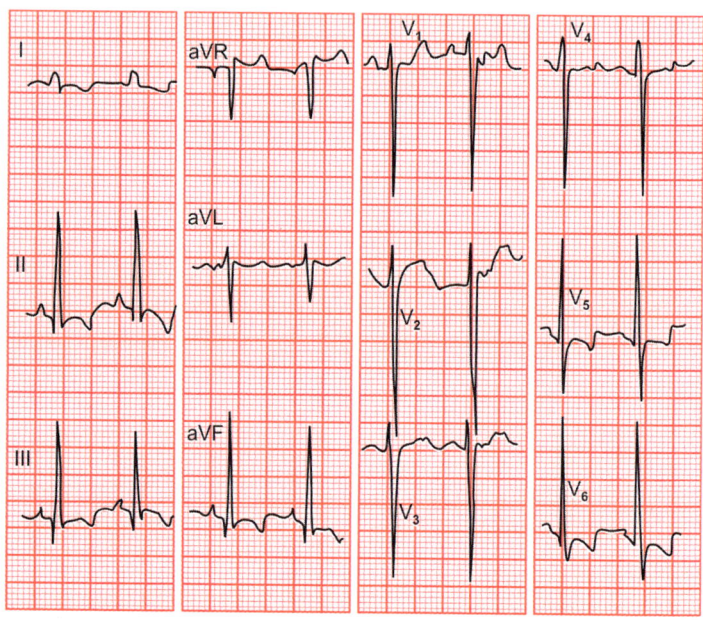

Interpretation

- Heart rate is about 107/min regular.
- Axis is normal.
- P-R interval normal
- The R wave is $V_5 + SV_1 = 40$ mm indicating left ventricular hypertrophy.
- There are Q wave in leads II, III, aVF and V_6. ST segment is depressed in leads I, II, III, aVF and V_4–V_6 indicating left ventricular strain.

ECG diagnosis: Left ventricular hypertrophy cause may be any. The clinical diagnosis of this patient was hypertorophic cardiomyopathy.

ECG 2

A young woman who appeared in medical board for examination for some reason. ECG was done which is displayed.

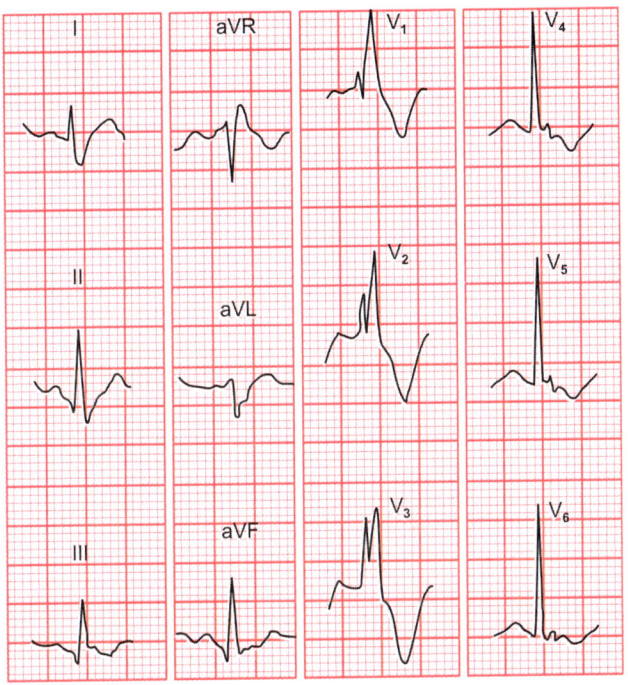

The ECG interpretation

1. Right axis deviation.
2. RSR' (rSR') pattern in leads V_1 and V_2 and M shaped R in V_3.
3. The duration of QRS is widened (> 0.12 sec).

ECG diagnosis: The findings suggest right bundle branch block which could be congenital or acquired (read the causes of RBBB).

ECG 3

A 60-year-old man was admitted with acute severe epigastric chest pain with profuse sweating. The ECG recorded in the casualty and emergency department is depicted.

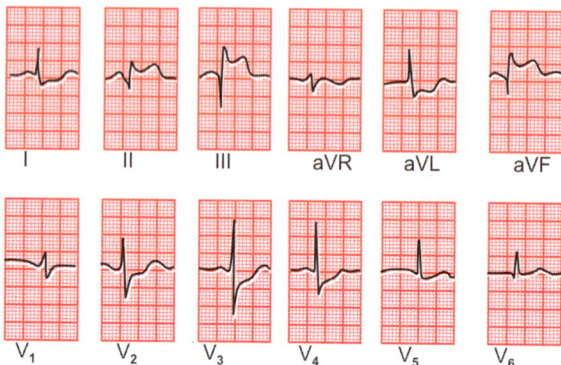

The ECG shows

i. Q waves and raised ST segment in inferior leads (II, III and aVF).

ii. There is reciprocal ST segment depression in leads, I, aVL V_2–V_5.

The ECG diagnosis is acute inferior wall infarction.

ECG 4

A woman landed in the medical outpatient department with palpitation. She was examined and ECG was taken (displayed).

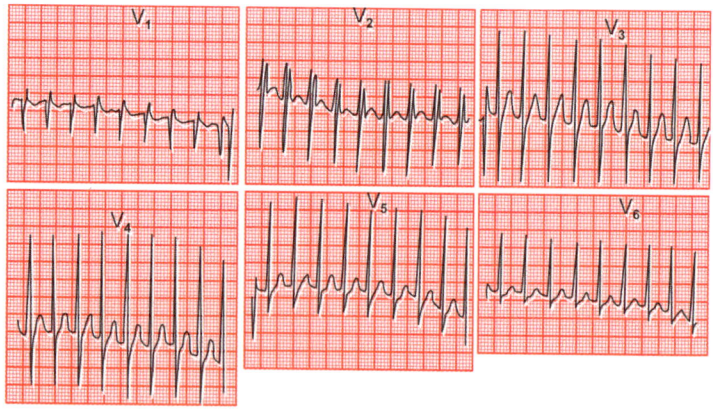

The ECG (leads V_1–V_6) shows

1. A regular narrow complex tachycardia at a rate of 200/min regular.

2. Cardiac axis cannot be commented.

3. No P wave is visible.
4. rsr' pattern is visible in leads V_1 and V_2 but duration is normal. This is incomplete bundle branch block.
5. ST segment and T waves are normal.

ECG diagnosis: Narrow QRS complex tachycardia probable paroxysmal supraventricular tachycardia.

ECG 5

A 45 years male complained of severe central chest pain at night. He was brought to the hospital in accidental emergency department. The ECG was taken (displayed).

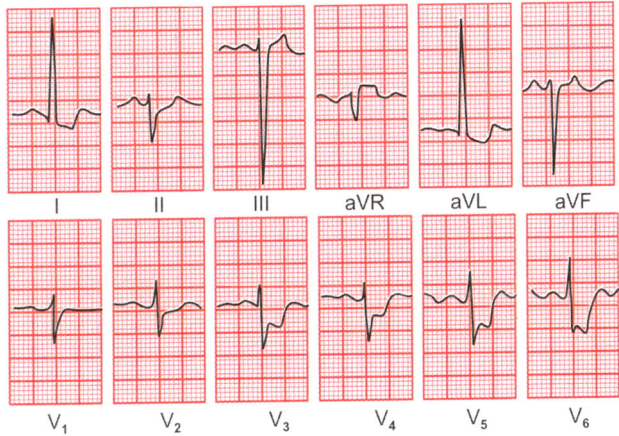

ECG Interpretation

• Left axis deviation (R wave in lead I and deep S wave in lead III).
• P wave and P-R interval normal.
• QRS complexes are normal and narrow.
• There is horizontal ST segment depression staying for more than 80 ms (2 small squares) in leads I, aVL and V_3 to V_6. The T wave is upright.
• There is no Q wave.

ECG diagnosis: The findings are suggestive of anterolateral ischaemia. To be correlated with the clinical findings.

Since the ECG findings correlated well with the clinical diagnosis of unstable angina or acute coronary syndrome, the patient was hospitalised for management.

ECG 6

A 20 years female complained of severe breathlessness, cough and haemoptysis. Examination reveals irregular pulse. BP was 110/70 mm right arm lying down. The lungs showed crackles. The JVP was raised. ECG was done (displayed).

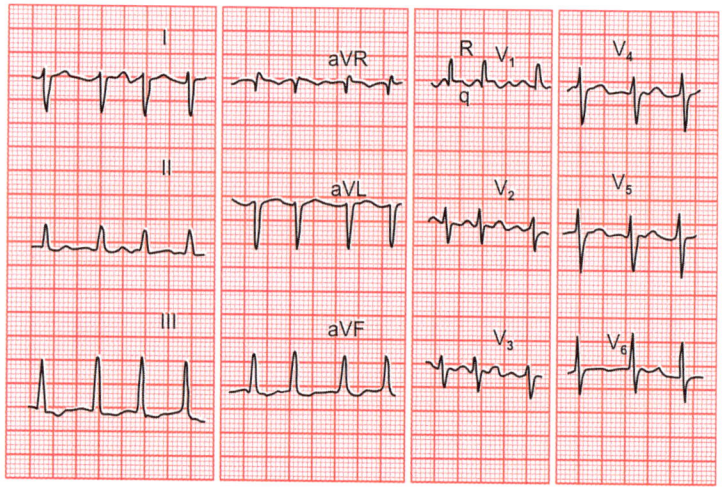

The ECG shows

  i. Right axis deviation (deep S wave in leads I and III).

  ii. Vertical heart position.

 iii. P waves not seen.

 iv. Heart rate is about 150/min R-R intervals are irregular.

  v. There is qR pattern in lead V_1 and R > S in lead V_2. There is clockwise rotation of heart (transition zone less in V_6). These findings suggest right ventricular hypertrophy.

 vi. There is ST depression and T inversion in lead V_1.

ECG diagnosis: Right ventricular hypertrophy with atrial fibrillation. The findings should be correlated with clinical diagnosis.

ECG 7

A young 40 years male had severe chest pain with nausea, vomiting and sweating. He was seen by the physician outside and was referred to the hospital for treatment. The ECG done at admission is displayed.

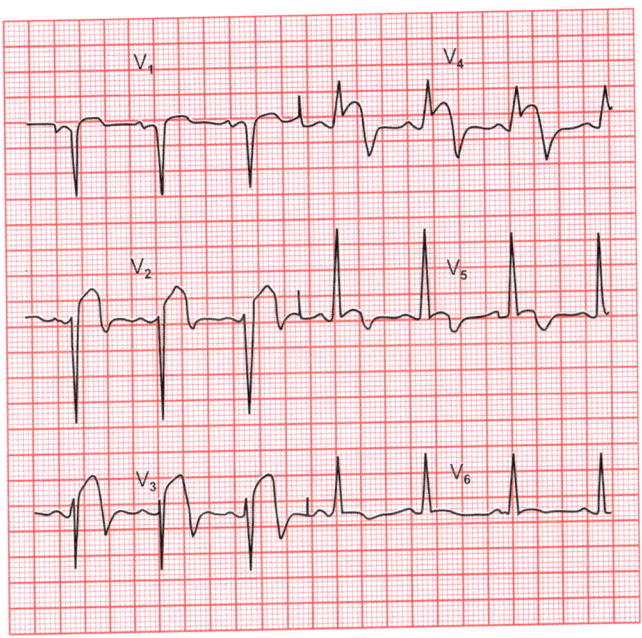

The chest leads (V_1–V_6) of the ECG show

- Axis cannot be commented.
- Heart rate is 80/min regular.
- P wave and P-R intervals are normal.
- No q wave seen.
- There is poor progression of R wave from V_1 to V_4
- There is ST elevation in leads V_1–V_5 with T wave inversion.

ECG diagnosis: The ECG is suggestive of ST elevation myocardial infarction. The findings correlated with the clinical diagnosis. Since the Q waves were not present the infarction was early, hence, patient was thrombolysed.

ECG 8

Read the rhythm strip lead II displayed.

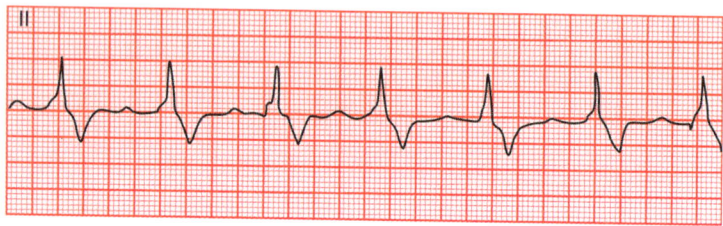

The rhythm strip of lead II ECG shows

- Axis cannot be commented.
- Rhythm is normal sinus.
- Heart rate is 75/min regular.
- P wave is normal.
- P-R interval is prolonged to 0.32 (8 small squares)
- QRS is narrow and normal.
- There is symmetric T wave inversion with sagging ST segment indicating ischaemia.

ECG diagnosis: ECG impression is 1st degree heart block. The cause may be inferior wall ischaemia because ST segment sagging with T wave inversion in lead II suggests inferior wall ischaemia. The full ECG or leads II, III, and aVF are needed to confirm the diagnosis.

ECG 9

A 50 years male was admitted with history of severe palpitation and breathlessness. Examination revealed poor volume pulse and BP was unrecordable. The ECG was done. The lead II is displayed.

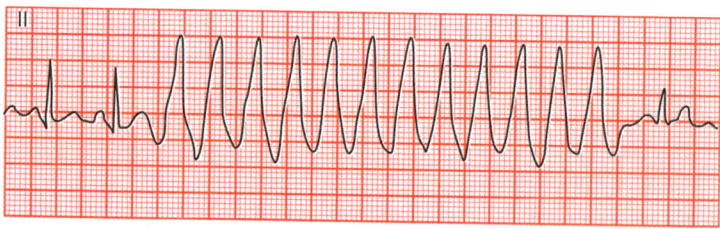

The lead II shows

i. Two normal narrow QRS complexes in the beginning are seen.

ii. There is a run of wide QRS complex tachycardia in the middle of the strip up to the end at a rate of 200/min regular.

iii. The last complex is again sinus (normal).

The ECG diagnosis is a run of ventricular tachycardia which is self-terminating.

ECG 10

The ECG lead V_1 was recorded from a patient who complained of vague chest discomfort and palpitation.

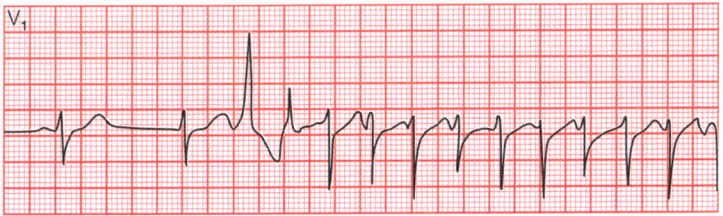

The lead V_1 shows

- First two complexes are normal.
- Third wide QRS complex is a ventricular extrasystole.
- The fourth narrow complex without P wave is again an atrial/supraventricular ectopic.
- This 4th supraventricular extrasystole triggered the narrow QRS complex tachycardia at the rate of 160/min.

The ECG diagnosis is ventricular and atrial ectopics with a run of paroxysmal supraventricular tachycardia.

ECG 11

A patient of mitral valve disease had breathlessness and palpitation. He was receiving digitalis also. The pulse was irregularly irregular. BP was 110/80 mm Hg. JVP was raised. Clinical examination revealed the findings of mitral stenosis. The ECG was done which showed right ventricular hypertrophy. The long lead II of the same patients is displayed.

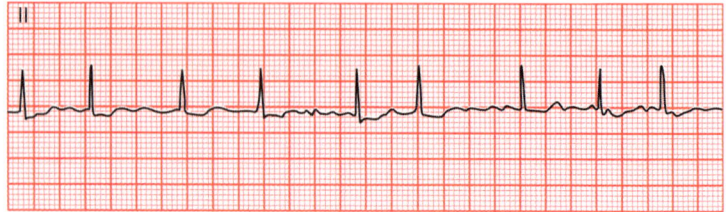

The lead II shows

- No visible P wave—the baseline is irregular and wavy due to small fibrillatory (f) waves.
- The R-R intervals are irregular from beat-to-beat.
- The QRS complexes are narrow.
- The ST segment is cup-shaped in the form of inverse tick mark sign, suggestive of digitalis effect/toxicity.

ECG diagnosis: The findings are suggestive of atrial fibrillation with digital effect/toxicity.

ECG 12

Read the rhythm strip (lead V_1) displayed.

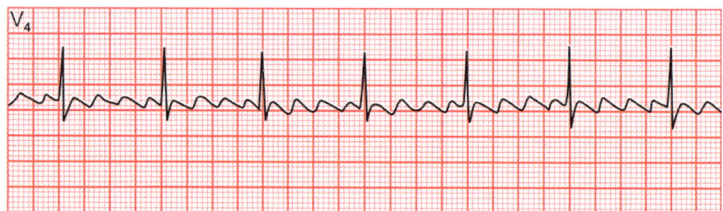

The rhythm strip lead V_4 shows

- No visible P wave. The baseline reveals saw-toothed appearance. The P waves are replaced by flutter (F) waves.
- In between R-R, there are four flutter (F) waves. Every 4th F wave is followed by a narrow QRS complex.
- There are narrow QRS complexes.
- The flutter rate is 300/min (1500 ÷ 5)
- The ventricular rate is 75/min.
- The conduction ratio between atria and ventricle is 4:1.

ECG diagnosis: The ECG shows atrial flutter with 4:1 conduction.

ECG 13

The ECG was taken from a patient of rheumatic heart disease. She was receiving digitalis. The pulse was irregular, hence, ECG was recorded and displayed.

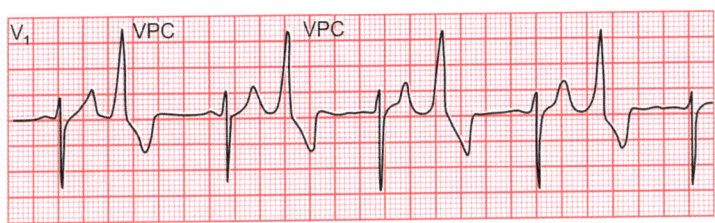

The ECG lead V₁ shows

- 1st complex (rS) in lead V_1 is normal. It is followed by a wide (> 0.14 sec) QRS complex with inverted T wave. This is a ventricular extrasystole.
- This pattern of one normal complex followed by an abnormal complex continues throughout the lead.
- An extrasystole following a normal QRS complex in a rhythmic fashion indicates ventricular bigeminy.

ECG diagnosis: Ventricular bigeminy.

Since the patient was receiving digitalis, hence, these extrasystoles are digitalis induced.

ECG 14

Read the rhythm strip lead I

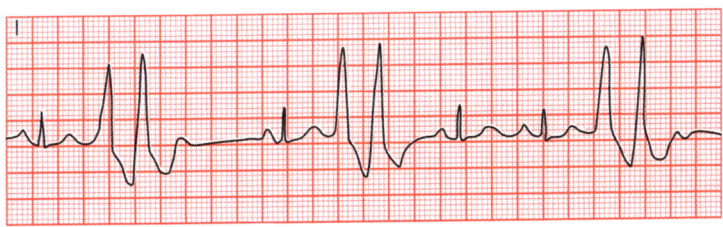

- The rhythm strip lead I shows a normal complex followed by a ventricular couplet (two ventricular extrasystoles in succession).
- Three ventricular couplets are seen.

ECG diagnosis: Frequent ventricular couplets. The ECG findings must be correlated to clinical diagnosis.

ECG 15

Read the rhythm strip lead V_3

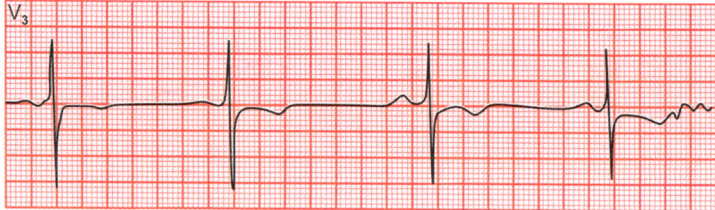

The ECG strip (V_3) shows

- Normal P waves.
- Regular sinus rhythm.
- Heart rate is 43/min regular.
- The QRS complexes are narrow.
- P-R interval is normal.

The ECG diagnosis is sinus bradycardia, cause may be any. Read the causes of sinus bradycardia.

ECG 16

A 25 years female presented with fever and acute chest pain of 5 days duration. The CVS examination revealed feeble heart sounds. The ECG was done (displayed).

The ECG shows

- Low voltage graph.
- Left axis deviation.
- Sinus tachycardia
- QRS complexes are wide (> 0.14 sec) slurred in V_5.
- QTc is prolonged.

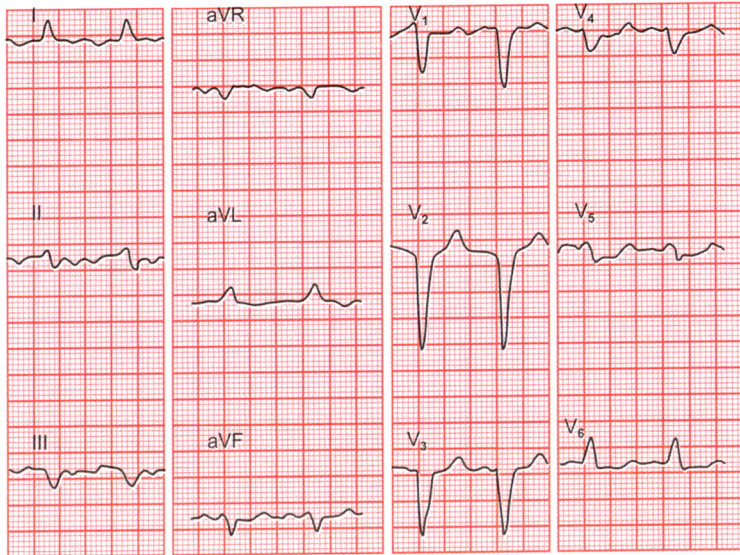

ECG diagnosis: The ECG shows LBBB pattern with prolonged QTc. Since, she has fever feeble heart sounds on auscultation and a low voltage graph, the underlying cause of ECG findings could be myocarditis.

ECG 17

Read the ECG lead II displayed

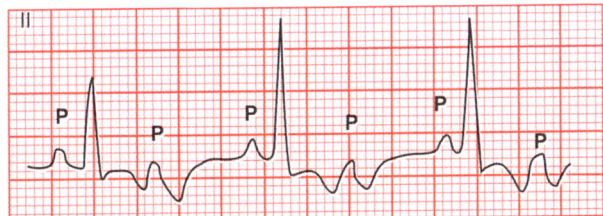

The ECG shows

i. Normal P waves and normal QRS complexes.

ii. There are more P waves than QRS.

iii. There are two P waves in between R-R interval. One P is blocked and the other P is conducted.

iv. The P-R interval of conducted P is fixed (0.14 sec).

ECG diagnosis: The ECG shows Mobitz type II second degree AV block with 2:1 conduction.

ECG 18

Read the ECG strip lead V₅ displayed

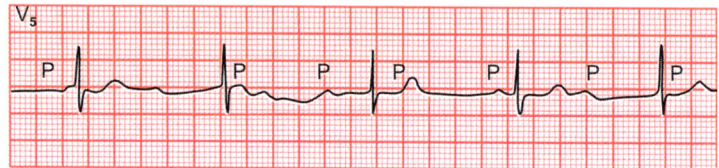

The ECG shows

- More P waves than QRS.
- P-R interval is not fixed.
- Heart rate is 56/min.
- P wave has no relation to QRS.
- The QRS is not wide, indicates infranodal block

ECG diagnosis: The ECG suggests complete heart block, cause of which may be any.

NB: The author now thinks that students will be able to interpret the ECG independently without any difficulty.

Index